# Miscarriage,
# Medicine &
# Miracles

# Miscarriage, Medicine & Miracles

## EVERYTHING YOU NEED TO KNOW ABOUT MISCARRIAGE

BRUCE K. YOUNG, M.D., F.A.C.O.G.,
AND AMY ZAVATTO

BANTAM BOOKS

MISCARRIAGE, MEDICINE & MIRACLES
A Bantam Book / May 2008

Published by
Bantam Dell
A Division of Random House, Inc.
New York, New York

Book design by Steve Kennedy
Illustrations by Sun Han

Bantam Books is a registered trademark of Random House, Inc., and the
colophon is a trademark of Random House, Inc.

Library of Congress Cataloging-in-Publication Data
Young, Bruce, M.D.
Miscarriage, medicine & miracles : everything you need to know
about miscarriage / Bruce Young and Amy Zavatto.
p.   cm.
ISBN 978-0-553-80550-5 (hardcover)
1. Miscarriage—Popular works.   I. Zavatto, Amy.   II. Title.
III. Title: Miscarriage, medicine and miracles.
RG648.Y68 2008
618.3'92—dc22        2007048179

Printed in the United States of America
Published simultaneously in Canada

www.bantamdell.com

10 9 8 7 6 5 4 3 2 1
BVG

This book is dedicated to my wonderful wife, Phyllis, who has been an inspiration and an example of the best a woman can be; to my loving daughters, Kathryn and Caroline; to Robby, Alison, and Zachy; and to all the women who have been my friends and patients, from whom I have learned so much.

— Bruce Young

For Dan, with all my love.

— Amy Zavatto

# ACKNOWLEDGMENTS

Both authors would like to thank the dazzling, judicious, and generally wonderful Joy Tutela for making this book happen, and Lissette Quinones, for her tireless efforts and constant, lovely smile.

Also, we would like to give a big thank-you to the great crew at Bantam, particularly Julie Will, for signing us up; Nita Taublib, for believing in the project; and Danielle Perez, for shepherding us through to the end.

Amy would also like to thank:
- Michael Zavatto, Linda Zavatto, and Laura Zavatto for loving me so much.
- The incredible, invaluable gold mine of friends I am lucky enough to have. You have each showed me such concern and love through this plight, but in particular I would like to tip my hat to Tamar Smith, Michele Morcey, Amy Bryant, Elizabeth Goodman Artis, and Patty Fiorenza, who went over and above the call of duty. Don't know where I'd be without you.
- Gary Karshmer for keeping me sane.
- Bonnie and Richard Gabor for encouraging us to take a seat in Bruce Young's office in the first place—I wouldn't be writing this without you.

# CONTENTS

~~~~~~~~~~~~~~~~~~~~~~~~~~~~~~~~~~~~~~~~~~~~~~~~~~~~~~~~~~~

# INTRODUCTION

One in four pregnant women in the United States will miscarry during pregnancy. It's an astoundingly large number—one that most women do not learn until they are sitting in a paper gown in their obstetrician's office, hearing the heartbreaking news about their pregnancy loss for the first time.

It is a fact that I, as an ob/gyn and as a specialist in high-risk pregnancy at New York University Medical Center, know well; and one that my co-author Amy Zavatto, a New York journalist, had to learn like the rest of those 25 to 30 percent of pregnant women: in a paper gown in another doctor's office.

Possibly more shocking than the high number of miscarriages that occur each year is the dearth of information available to women and their spouses on the topic, most of which is woefully out of date or deals simply (and often inadequately) with the emotional side of the issue. Even more surprising may be the response many women receive from their own trusted physicians—doctors who thrive when their patients have healthy pregnancies, but who, when it comes to dealing with multiple miscarriages, give the often-heard and unsatisfying response, "It's nature's way."

In fact, a patient isn't considered at "high risk" for multiple miscarriages until she has experienced three subsequent lost pregnancies, forcing those who want to become parents to roll the proverbial dice over and over until the average ob/gyn (and, of course, their health-insurance providers) will give them more than a sidelong glance. Because most physicians won't raise a red flag after one or two lost pregnancies, the statistics for recurrent miscarriage remain the same until the patient has gone through a third harrowing lost pregnancy. That, according to present statistics, raises the rate of recurrence to 28 percent. It is only then that the patient receives further testing, investigation, and special consideration from an average ob/gyn. If she wants to see a specialist prior to this and buck the medical standards in place, it's her dime. Or her risk.

When Amy and I met, we learned that we had more in common besides our doctor/patient relationship; we wanted to fix what was wrong. During my forty years in practice, I knew that thorough testing and diagnosis were key components often missing for many of my patients prior to arriving in my office. I've encountered countless patients like Amy, who had experienced miscarriages and who came to me with the two gnawing questions that plague every woman who miscarries; questions I had heard time and time again:

"Why did this happen to me?"
"What can I do to prevent it the next time?"

These unhappy women need to have those questions answered. And women who are pregnant, or thinking about becoming pregnant, and are worried about miscarrying need to have their issues addressed, too.

In this book, we take an exhaustive look into not just the basics of pregnancy, miscarriage, and what to expect when it occurs, but the specific medical reasons that address *why* women miscarry. It presents an in-depth look into the causes of miscarriage as no other book has done before. Using individual clinical cases from my practice, each chapter highlights a particular reason for pregnancy loss (from diabetes, to genetics, to hormonal deficiencies, to auto-immune disorder, and a host of other issues) and explains why and how miscarriage occurs in that particular case. All the case histories are true, but I have changed the names and some non-medical details to avoid anyone being identified in order to protect my patients' privacy.

This book provides illustrations of female reproductive function to clearly demonstrate where and how the problem occurs, and describes the vital diagnostic tools, as well as the approaches to treatment and prevention, using the most up-to-date information and technology.

It's a book that should have been written a long time ago. According to the American College of Obstetricians and Gynecologists, a definite cause for miscarriage—or, as it is not-so-gently referred to in the medical field, spontaneous abortion—can be found in only 50 percent of diagnosed cases. This is disheartening information if you've been through it and have come up empty-handed and empty-cradled, over and over again. When a woman miscarries, it leaves her in a distorted state of self-accusation and blame. It's a bit like having your house robbed again and again despite taking all the proper precautions—you think you're doing all the right things to protect yourself (in the case of pregnancy, eating well and steering clear of risky foods, taking prenatal vitamins, being cautious about over-the-top physical exertion), but then, inexplicably, it happens again.

I believe that 50 percent statistic can be improved enormously if we physicians approach miscarriage the way we would approach disease: by undertaking an extensive diagnostic evaluation as the first step.

When a woman becomes pregnant, there are mountains of information exploding from bookshelves on pregnancy and childbirth—pregnancy books; baby-name books; magazines of the same ilk; catalogues showing the latest in baby-room décor, maternity wear, or mommy-on-the-go gadgets; even Web sites that will calculate a pregnancy day-by-day.

It's a different story for miscarriage. When a woman loses a pregnancy, there is a huge, gaping hole where, for her prior condition, there were tons of facts and support. Nobody talks about miscar-riage. Nobody compares notes. There is no *Girlfriends' Guide to Dealing with Miscarriage* to bestow helpful tidbits of information on what is going on with a woman's body and how this might affect her physically and emotionally. To tell her what the common follow-up procedure to miscarriage—a D&C—is like. To tell her the particular reasons why she may miscarry or what tests can give her this specific information. To tell her what can be done to prevent it next time.

It seems like a painful, seemingly clandestine club to which thousands of women gain admittance every year without asking for or desiring membership. Amy found when she revealed to friends or co-workers that she had experienced multiple miscar-riages, it was as if she'd given the secret handshake: suddenly, she was privy to information about an acquaintance's sister or cousin, a co-worker's daughter, or even, sometimes, the loss experienced by a friend.

We found that there are a few different issues working against Amy and her husband: a general lack of progesterone during the first trimester of pregnancy (easily corrected), a genetic disorder called monosomy 21 from a balanced translocation (less easily cor-rected, but possible to work around through IVF), and age. These problems will be discussed in detail in this book, as well as many others. Her fifth and last miscarriage was age related, squarely fit-ting into the over-35 statistics of Amy's age group. Amy sometimes jokes with me that she and her husband are the poster children of bad percentages, that small X percent for whom things do not go as planned. But as much as she uses humor as a deflective shield and soother for awkward conversations or questions, she tells me the real truth. Amy feels perched in a terrified sort of limbo. "The more I sit and wait," she tells me, "the more keenly aware I become that I'm allowing time to make the decision for me."

As an ob/gyn, I have devoted my life to caring for women like my co-author. I have shared their experiences of loss and joy, especially the feelings surrounding childbearing. As a husband and father of daughters, I have lived a different role from physician alone. For many years, I have thought about writing more than a scientific text to help women afflicted by miscarriage. When Amy and I met as doctor and patient, the subject came up again and there was a meeting of minds. This book is the result.

It's a lonely plight, but miscarriage certainly doesn't have to be the walk in the dark that so many women experience. This book doesn't just shine a strong, bright light on the reasons for miscarriage and how to go on to a successful pregnancy; it gives the woman who experiences multiple miscarriages something that she might have lost along the way: hope.

# section one

~~~~~~~~~~~~~~~~~~~~~~~~~~~~~~~~~~~~~~~~~~

## THE BASICS

# one

## PREPARING FOR PREGNANCY:
## UNDERSTANDING YOUR BODY

~~~~~~~~~~~~~~~~~~~~~~~~~~~~~~~~~~~~~~~~~~~~~~~~~~~~~~~~~~~~~

NEWLYWEDS DIANA AND GREG STARTED TO THINK ABOUT having children within the first year they tied the knot. Now 25, Diana had been my patient since she was a teenager. At her routine visit six months before, I congratulated her on her recent marriage and her new job as a fund-raiser for the university she'd attended as an undergrad. I suggested that she come in for a pre-pregnancy session and bring along her husband, Greg, an outgoing and friendly newspaper writer, to discuss pregnancy.

When I met Diana ten years ago, her mother had brought her to my office. She was 15 and had been complaining of abdominal pain, which was getting worse and worse. At first, she told me, the pain came and went, although it was sometimes severe, but lately it was nearly continuous and she could not function at all. That day in my office she said the pain was across her lower abdomen and came in waves, but was constant and worse on the right side. It had gotten so bad it was affecting not just her after-school soccer, but her academic work as well. Understandably, both Diana and her mom were anxious about this frightening problem.

I examined Diana and found her abdomen to be very tender. I did a sonogram, which showed me that she had an ovarian cyst, causing a twisted right ovary—immediate surgery was necessary to save her ovary. I performed **laparoscopic surgery,** removed the cyst, and was able to untwist the ovary and save it, preserving her fertility.

## laparoscopic surgery

Considered a minimally invasive procedure, laparoscopic surgery is performed by making several small incisions in the abdomen, usually one-half to one centimeter in length. An incision is made through the navel (although the incision may also be made just below the navel, I like to make it through the navel so the scar can't be seen). A thin, long tube called a laparoscope is inserted through the incision into the patient. A camera is attached to the outside of the laparoscope, enabling the surgeon to see inside the patient by viewing an image on a TV screen transmitted by the camera. Tiny instruments are then inserted through secondary incisions to perform the surgery.

Now, a decade later, Diana was ready to put that fertility to use. She and Greg were planning pregnancy in about four months, after she finished working on a particularly stressful fund-raiser for the university's capital endowment. I reviewed each of their medical histories and asked about their families to be sure that there were no hereditary problems or increased risk for miscarriage.

I examined Diana again and confirmed that there were no new findings and that she remained physically well. There was no residual scarring from her previous surgery; in fact, there were no visible scars from the laparoscopic surgery. Her fertility was not affected and she was in great shape to get pregnant.

Still, even with a clean bill of health there were some preliminary steps to be taken. I explained genetic screening to the couple and offered them our panel of blood tests for genetic diagnosis, best to be done at this time. I gave them my printed information for pregnant women, which contains answers to the most common questions and recommendations for nutrition and exercise, and describes normal changes in pregnancy. I began Diana on prenatal vitamins to be sure she had high levels in her body before she was pregnant. I explained the normal changes in pregnancy, what to expect, and what was not normal. I answered all the questions she and Greg had. Then I sent Diana for the standard blood tests for prenatal screening.

All Diana's tests were normal. She and Greg followed my advice about stopping the birth control pill and switched to condoms until they were ready to try for pregnancy. Five months later, they conceived. The following nine months were uneventful except at the very end, when labor started. Diana was at work, going over some photos of an event for a news release she'd just finished. She ignored the contractions, approved the final shot for the piece—and then realized she was in the middle of her own newsworthy story.

She quickly called me, Greg, and then a car service. Her water broke as she came through the front door of NYU Medical Center where Greg was waiting. I met them on the elevator, and I whisked her into a delivery room.While Greg was changing to join us, Diana began to push. Three more pushes and I gave Diana and Greg the news they'd been waiting for—an 8 lb 4 oz boy named Stephen.

## HOW DO YOU BECOME PREGNANT?

I reviewed birth control methods with Diana and Greg. I advised her to stop the birth control pill she'd been using for three months before trying to conceive and switch to condoms or a diaphragm to avoid any possible increased risk of miscarriage.

### birth control and miscarriage

There is thought to be an increased risk of miscarriage with pregnancy right after stopping the pill. The reasons are possibly slow re-growth of the lining of the womb so that it is not ready to support a pregnancy, and irregular return of ovulation, which may not synchronize with the growth of the lining of the womb. Both of those problems may prevent normal implantation (attachment of the fertilized egg to the wall of the uterus) and inadequate development of the placenta leading to miscarriage.

Of course, you don't need to get "the talk" from me, but you'd be surprised at how even the most well-educated, well-informed people can still be a little bit in the dark on how, step-by-step, pregnancy occurs. Even if you've got the procedure down pat, it is truly an amazing occurrence and one of the phenomenal things a woman's body can do.

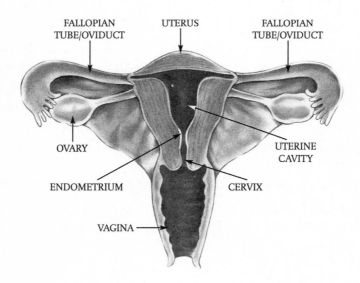

The **uterus** consists of the cervix, which is attached to the top of the vagina, and the corpus or "body." The cervix allows fluid to *leave* the uterus and enter the vagina, as in menstruation, or fluid from the vagina to *enter* the uterus, such as seminal fluid, which carries the sperm into the uterus for fertilization and pregnancy.

The **cervix** is the "mouth" of the uterus (or womb) and the "body" is the upper part, which is where the pregnancy usually forms.

---

## cervix

The part of the uterus (womb) that protrudes into the top of the vagina and has an opening into the uterus. It is often referred to as the mouth of the womb.

---

## uterus

The female reproductive organ to which the fallopian tubes and cervix are attached. Also called the womb, it carries the pregnancy.

---

Fertilization occurs when the sperm enter the uterus and then swim up to meet the egg, which was released by one of the two ovaries. This meeting usually happens in the oviduct (**fallopian tube**) or "tube," which sweeps up the egg and moves it toward the uterus after it is released from the ovary (**ovulation**). After sperm and egg meet (fertilization), the fertilized egg continues down the tube and attaches to the wall of the uterus (**implantation**), where it forms the **placenta** (afterbirth) and the embryo that becomes the baby.

---

## placenta

The afterbirth, which is an organ of fetal origin that grows into the mother's uterine wall for its blood supply and provides oxygen and nutrition to the fetus while removing fetal carbon dioxide and products of fetal metabolism.

### fallopian tubes

Also called oviducts, these are the flexible, moving structures that carry the released eggs, or ova, from the ovaries to the uterus.

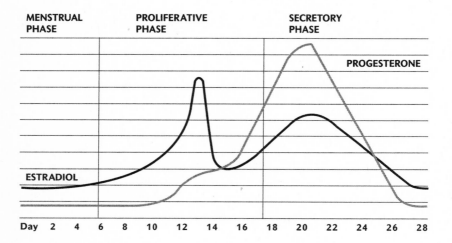

### ovulation

The midway point during the menstrual cycle when a mature egg, or ovum, is released from an ovary and sent down the fallopian tube (oviduct) toward the uterus to await fertilization. If fertilization does not occur, the egg will be absorbed. Although most menstrual cycles are based on a 28-day calendar, many women have shorter or longer cycles, and thus ovulation can occur earlier or later than the standard midpoint of day 14 to 16. Every month the cycle is started by hormones that stimulate up to 20 of the 300,000 or so eggs stored in your ovaries. Usually, only one egg develops enough to respond to the hormonal trigger to ovulate, while the others break down and get absorbed. Once the egg and sperm meet in the oviduct and unite in fertilization, the embryo begins to form as it journeys to the uterus. That trip takes about three days and then the embryo attaches itself to the wall of the uterus. This is implantation, as the embryo buries itself in the lining tissues of the uterus and is nourished there.

## implantation

A process by which the embryo buries itself in the lining of the uterus, the endometrium.

## PRE-PREGNANCY TESTING

Earlier in this chapter, I briefly mentioned that there were tests I advised Diana to undergo before getting pregnant, as well as recommendations I gave her for staying pregnant for the full nine months. Let's take a closer look at those now.

After I had completed their medical and family histories and examined Diana, I sent the couple for genetics testing. This has become a fairly standard routine today even in the absence of a significant medical history for two reasons:

1. There are many tests available to evaluate a person's genetic history and recognize any possible genetic problems *before* the pregnancy occurs. In this way the problems that might lead to miscarriage can be detected, and possibly avoided, particularly since 80 percent of miscarriages are related to a genetic abnormality.
2. Each couple may have genetic factors that bear on the outcome of pregnancy and the risk for specific diseases as well. Now that we are able to know the human genome (the DNA code that describes every individual's makeup), soon

we will be able to calculate risks for some diseases and for certain pregnancy problems.

I also ordered a number of other tests for Diana. The standard tests that I prefer to obtain before pregnancy are as follows:

1. *Blood type and Rh factor.* This test is performed to detect blood incompatibilities that could lead to pregnancy loss. (See Chapter 19.)
2. *Complete blood count.* This test detects anemias and low platelet counts, as well as high white blood cell count to look for infections, which are associated with increased risk for miscarriage and pregnancy complications.
3. *Specific tests for infections with possible pregnancy risks.* I recommend being tested for toxoplasmosis, cytomegalovirus, rubella (German measles), varicella (chicken pox), syphilis (the test is called RPR, or rapid plasma reagin), and the most common form of hepatitis, hepatitis B (the test is called the hepatitis B surface antigen). For some patients at increased risk based on their medical history of multiple sexual partners and unprotected sex, other tests may be ordered to look for sexually transmitted diseases, such as chlamydia and gonorrhea.
4. *Thyroid tests.* Low or high thyroid activity can be related to miscarriage, so I order the following tests: TSH (thyroid-stimulating hormone), free thyroxine, and total triiodothyronine. (See Chapter 15.)
5. *Urinalysis and urine culture.* I order these tests to confirm normal kidney function and the absence of chronic urinary infection, since both of these can lead to pregnancy loss. (See Chapter 14.)

If there is a history of previous miscarriage I will add specific tests looking for vaginal bacteria and mycoplasmas (a type of infecting agent that is a rare kind of bacteria-like organism) and other various tests based on the patient's specific history.

If all the results are normal, then I get to the part of the discussion that inevitably leads to questions throughout a woman's entire pregnancy: the plan for diet, exercise, and travel. I discuss many of the myths and much false information about each of these topics in Chapter 7, but right now we're going to lay the groundwork for a healthy pregnancy—yours.

## DIET AND HEALTH

In general, diet guidelines are widely applicable. Good sense goes a long way, but of course there's always room for doubt and questions with so much information (and misinformation) out there on the topic. Just as you learned in school, a healthy diet should follow the FDA food pyramid. Additionally, prenatal vitamins that contain pregnancy-appropriate amounts of folic acid should be taken

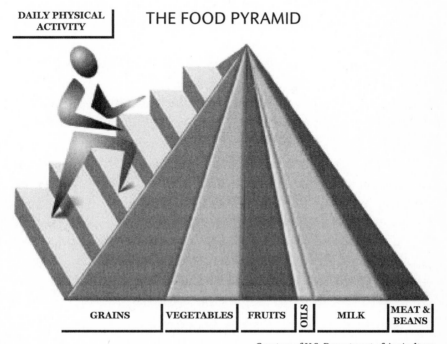

**DAILY PHYSICAL ACTIVITY**

## THE FOOD PYRAMID

| GRAINS | VEGETABLES | FRUITS | OILS | MILK | MEAT & BEANS |

*Courtesy of U.S. Department of Agriculture*

starting at least one month before conception. Although one of the best things nature does is to provide for the baby's nutrition by allowing it to extract what it needs from the pregnant woman, dietary folic acid needs to be supplemented to be sure that there is enough to prevent birth defects. Enriched grain foods like cereals, breads, and pastas are particularly good dietary sources of folic acid for pregnancy.

Other supplements may be of benefit, like calcium, iron, and omega-3 fatty acids, since they may be lacking in the mother-to-be's diet and the fetus also needs them. (See Chapter 2.) However, excess amounts of dietary supplements may be harmful and you should avoid taking extra supplements beyond your doctor's recommendations. For example, vitamins A and D tend to accumulate rather than be excreted by the body and they may cause miscarriage or fetal abnormalities when taken in excess. If you've been taking a regular multivitamin daily, do not worry. The amounts of these vitamins are well within the normal, appropriate range for a healthy adult. This goes for your prenatal vitamins, too, once you start taking them.

"Natural" supplements advertised as dietary supplements, derived from natural sources and used in different cultures, have become extremely popular in the last few decades. However, most are not tested scientifically and the possible risks and benefits are not accurately known. Different minerals, botanicals, plant extracts, and pills from complementary and alternative medical sources are classified as nutrients rather than drugs. Because of that, they are not required to meet FDA standards for safety and efficacy. If you are taking any supplements at all, they should be used only after discussion with your doctor or midwife. Also, higher than required levels of vitamins besides A and D may have negative effects when they interact in pregnancy, which is a field just beginning to be studied. For example, excess calcium can block absorption of iron and lead to anemia. Excess folic acid can interfere with vitamin

$B_{12}$ function, and excess tea drinking can also block some aspects of iron absorption. In other words, more is not better—and it can be worse. Our understanding of nutrition in pregnancy is quite limited, so the best advice for preventing pregnancy loss is a healthy diet with prenatal vitamins with folic acid as prescribed. Remember, over-the-counter non-prescribed supplements may not be helpful and could be harmful.

## PHYSICAL ACTIVITY DURING PREGNANCY

Being fit during pregnancy is important and will aid in keeping you and your baby healthy. With that said, exercise in early pregnancy should be limited to about two-thirds of what you were doing before you became pregnant. Once you are past the first three months it can be increased based on your caregiver's recommendation. Medical literature does not show a relationship between exercise and miscarriage. However, most women are easily tired in early pregnancy as the body adjusts to the hormonal changes. Adequate rest is just as valuable as adequate exercise, and you definitely should not begin training for a marathon or a triathlon during pregnancy. Unless there is a specific problem, normal exercise with limited stress on your body is generally recommended. Good examples are swimming, jogging, yoga, and aerobics.

Sexual activity has not been shown to cause miscarriage, but has been associated with preterm labor. Unless your caregiver advises against it, your usual sexual activity is fine in pregnancy. However, certain conditions are associated with miscarriage and will require abstaining from sexual intercourse. These include vaginal bleeding, painful intercourse, cramping, ruptured membranes, and a low-lying placenta on sonograms.

## ON YOUR WAY

Preparing for a healthy pregnancy is important, but still you may well be wondering: "Okay, I know what to do to be healthy, but

what risk factors may be present that could cause me to miscarry?"
In the absence of any specific diagnosis or known disease, there are
some risks that we can identify:

1.  Three consecutive miscarriages
2.  Obesity
3.  Previous fertility treatments, especially in vitro
    fertilization (IVF)
4.  The woman's age over 35
5.  An active infection in pregnancy
6.  Smoking during pregnancy
7.  Consuming alcohol on a daily basis during pregnancy
8.  Cocaine or amphetamine use during pregnancy
9.  Malnutrition or severe anorexia
10. Irregular ovulation
11. Vaginal bleeding
12. Rupture of membranes

These may seem like a lot of things to worry about, but several
items on the list are within your control and can easily be avoided.
However, other items, like previous fertility treatment, age, or
three consecutive miscarriages, are truly beyond your control. But
take heart: most of these factors can be dealt with *before* becoming pregnant and with proper care during pregnancy. With
pre-conceptional counseling, close evaluation in early pregnancy,
laboratory tests such as the ones I recommended earlier, and ultrasound studies as I've described, the large majority of women can
avoid miscarriage even with known risk factors. A normal pregnancy with a healthy baby are the expected outcomes when you are
expecting. Even high-risk women can have a healthy baby—I've
delivered an awful lot of them.

# two

## NUTRITION AND PREGNANCY: FEEDING THE BABY

~~~~~~~~~~~~~~~~~~~~~~~~~~~~~~~~~~~~~~~~~~~~~~~~~~~~~

HEALTHY NUTRITION IS IMPORTANT THROUGHOUT LIFE for men and women. The adage "You are what you eat" is not exactly right, but it is close. I would say it really is "You are what you make of what you eat"—and in pregnancy, you are making a baby in addition to maintaining your own health.

There have always been culturally different beliefs about foods and eating in pregnancy. In ancient China, eating goat was thought to produce a stubborn child, while one African tribe says that only cow's blood and milk are appropriate nutrition. In the 1940s and 1950s in the United States, a proper diet for pregnancy restricted calories, red meat, and salt in order to prevent preeclampsia and excessively large babies. Today, we know this is wrong.

The understanding of clinical nutrition is still limited, but we have better insight today than a generation ago because we continue to study nutrition in a scientific context. In order to understand our dietary needs, we should know some basics. Nutrition provides energy for the body to carry out its functions; ingredients for the body to build its structures, grow, and develop; and substances to help the chemical reactions that sustain these functions. The macronutrients are the proteins, carbohydrates, and fats in food, and the micronutrients are the vitamins and minerals that are important contributors to these processes.

Proper nutrition for pregnancy begins in the months before conception. Except in cases of severe starvation, miscarriage is unlikely due to under-nutrition or malnutrition, as far as we know today. However, birth defects, low birth weight, brain dysfunction, and long-term illness in adults, such as diabetes, heart disease, and hypertension, are associated with fetal malnutrition. Before becoming pregnant, every woman should have a visit with her obstetrician/gynecologist to discuss planning for pregnancy, including nutritional counseling. Pre-pregnancy weight should be considered and a plan for appropriate weight gain discussed. Women of average weight and height should expect to gain about 25 pounds with a dietary intake of around 36 calories per kg, which is about 2,200 calories per day.

Of course, this visit is an opportunity to ask questions, not only about nutrition, but any other concerns that you may have. This is when to have your doctor or midwife discuss vaccinations and medical problems, smoking, alcohol, drugs and toxins, and to send you for prenatal testing. At this visit, you and your health-care provider should discuss which nutrients, and how much of each of them, you should have based on your own dietary preferences and the recommendations of the Institute of Medicine, the National Institutes of Health, or the American College of Obstetricians and Gynecologists. They are similar but not exactly alike so you can use them as guidelines.

The healthy-diet food pyramid is available on page 11 and can be varied within wide limits. Keep in mind that you have an increased need for calories in order to supply your growing baby with the nutrition he or she (or they) will need. The basic nutritional requirements of pregnancy are as follows:

- *More protein!* You will need a minimum of 100 g daily, so vegetarian diets need to be adjusted for this increase. Meat, fish, poultry, beans, cheese, milk, and eggs are your best sources of protein. For example, either six ounces of meat or four cups of cottage cheese would do it for a day.

- *Carbohydrates and fiber.* In general, daily carbohydrates should include two cups of fruit and two and a half cups of vegetables, three or more ounces of whole grains, and another three ounces from enriched grain products, based on the United States Department of Agriculture food pyramid. They are also your best source of fiber, which is needed more in pregnancy.

- *Healthy fats.* Fats should make up less than 30 percent of calories, keeping cholesterol to under 300 mg a day and trans fats and saturated fats to 10 percent or less of total fats. You should try to get your fats from fish, nuts, olive oil, fish oils, and foods that are especially rich in omega-3 fatty acids.

- *Dairy.* Milk is a good source of many nutrients, and three or more glasses a day is another excellent choice. Yogurts and sour cream are similar. The low-fat varieties are fine for milk and milk products. Artificial sweeteners that are believed to be safe are NutraSweet and Splenda, the ones in the blue and the yellow packets. The saccharine in Sweet'N Low is an artificial substance believed to be safe also. NutraSweet is aspartame, an amino acid derivative that can be used by the body. Splenda is made from a sugar-like substance, sucralose, which is broken down by the body. Saccharine is the only truly foreign substance. None of them have been fully tested in pregnant women, but none have been found to cause miscarriage. Consult your doctor to decide about artificial sweeteners in pregnancy.

- *Lots of water!* You need more water when you're pregnant, so be sure to keep a bottle anywhere that makes it convenient for you to pick it up and drink about eight glasses a day. You need water to make new blood for mother and baby, amniotic fluid, and to increase kidney function throughout pregnancy.

The micronutrients, which are the vitamins and minerals in your food, should be adequate before starting the pregnancy. Practically speaking, your daily diet should include all of these, but there is so much variation in what people eat that a **supplement** is usually prescribed before pregnancy to ensure a healthy start.

---

### supplement
An additional nutrient that may be added to your usual diet.

---

Most important of these micronutrients is folic acid. When you are preparing for pregnancy and during your first trimester, 400 to 800 mcg daily is the recommended amount because it has been shown to reduce the risk of fetal abnormalities. These include neural tube defects, such as spina bifida, an opening in the spine, and hydrocephaly, water on the brain, as well as some malformations of the fetal heart. It is estimated that taking a higher dose, 4 or 5 mg per day of folic acid, before conception and in early pregnancy could decrease the frequency of neural tube defects by 82 percent in high-risk women. They are those for whom there has been a previous fetal malformation, or women who are in an older age group or of Irish and English descent.

Folic acid (along with vitamin $B_{12}$ and iron) is needed to prevent the mom from getting anemic and to build the baby's blood as well. Also, according to studies summarized by the March of Dimes, taking the **recommended dietary allowance (RDA)** of 400 micrograms of folic acid could decrease the occurrence of neural tube defects in America by 36 to 85 percent if made available to the entire pregnant population. There are other data suggesting that the risk of fetal heart defects can be reduced by folic acid, as well. Since humans absorb only about 50 percent of the folic acid in food, the United States government requires that flour be fortified with folic acid. That means that breads, cereal, and most grain-based products are enriched with folic acid. When you buy noodles, spaghetti, breads, and cereals, look for the word "enriched" to be sure that the folic acid has been added. Sometimes, the word **fortified** is used instead, and they mean the same thing. Whole-grain foods have more vitamins and folic acid than milled grain products to start with, but all should be enriched with additional folic acid. Recent studies suggest that 800 micrograms might be better in early pregnancy, possibly due to poor absorption. You should ask your doctor for a recommended prenatal vitamin prescription.

---

## recommended dietary allowance (rda)

The average daily intake that is sufficient to meet the nutritional requirements of nearly all healthy persons in each age and gender group, as well as in pregnancy.

---

## fortified

The addition of essential nutrients to a food, regardless of whether that nutrient is normally contained in the food, for the purpose of improving the diet.

---

There are other supplements you need, too, including:

- *Vitamin $B_{12}$*, 4 mcg per day, to prevent anemia and nerve injury.

    The other B vitamins like $B_6$, biotin, and riboflavin are present in varying doses in most prenatal vitamins, but in excess in most American diets.

- *Vitamin D*, 400 IU to 800 IU per day. Calcium is needed for the teeth and bones, and vitamin D in 400 IU to 800 IU per day amounts is important for absorbing the calcium into the teeth and bones. Too much vitamin D can be harmful, however, as can too much vitamin A, causing fetal abnormalities, although these are not usually associated with miscarriage. So, more is not better, and you should stay within the RDA amounts for pregnancy and not exceed the **tolerable upper intake level (UL)**.
- *Vitamins C and E*. These nutrients are frequently removed from food when it is processed. Foods that are boiled, canned, and preserved are often low in these nutrients. Fresh fruits and vegetables have lots of these, and the RDA is only 100 mg per day.
- *Iron*. A daily dose of ferrous or chelated iron equal to 27 to 45 mg will be absorbed well enough during pregnancy to cover the increased needs of a pregnant woman and her baby. Iron stores are often low in women because of the iron lost with menstrual bleeding and not replaced by a diet rich in meats and leafy-green vegetables, like spinach and kale. The mother's blood volume and red blood cell mass must increase substantially, and the baby's blood also has to be made from this iron source.
- *Calcium* is a necessary nutrient for strong teeth and bones (for both you and the baby!). Fifteen hundred mg per day should be enough.
- *Zinc* seems to be beneficial for the immune system and may be helpful in preventing preterm labor, with an RDA about 15 mg a day.
- *Magnesium* helps absorb calcium, and may also help avoid preterm birth. The RDA is about 300 mg per day.
- *Iodine* is needed for development of the baby's thyroid gland, but here again, too much may cause an abnormality

in the fetal thyroid function or even in the mother's. Only trace amounts, about 150 micrograms, are needed.

So, prenatal vitamins containing all of these and vitamin C, which helps to absorb the iron, are usually prescribed and will not exceed the **tolerable upper intake level** in this dosage.

---

## tolerable upper intake level (ul)

The maximum amount of a nutrient that can be taken on a daily basis, which poses no risk of an adverse effect on the health of the mother or baby.

---

In pregnancy, we want the micronutrients dose to be just right; after all, they are *micro*nutrients, needed in small amounts only. In fact, there are many other micronutrients needed in only trace amounts, such as manganese, copper, strontium, chromium, and molybdenum, which are present in food and water, so that supplements with them are seldom necessary.

Recently, nutritional research has found a powerful relationship between omega-3 fatty acids and development of the brain and eyesight in young children. There appears to be a clear relationship between good vision and cognitive skills in children exposed to omega-3s compared with other children of the same age and socioeconomic background. The result is a number of prenatal vitamins with omega-3s added or sold with a second tablet containing the omega-3s, docosahexaenoic acid (DHA) and eicosapentaenoic acid (EPA). These are usually supplied in a suggested dose of 300 to 500 mcg per day. This is an example of a nutraceutical with a proven benefit. Many others are sold without proof of any benefit despite extensive advertising of their value, both in pregnancy and in the non-pregnant state. You should not take these **nutraceuticals** without first consulting your doctor or midwife.

nutraceutical

A food or part of a food or food supplement that may provide medical or general health benefits. It is often a natural product, such as garlic, or it may be a specific component of a food, such as the omega-3s in fish oil, or it may be a natural product with no specific basis for activity as a food supplement.

Eating properly in pregnancy can be a challenge in each trimester. In the first three months, many women have nausea and loss of appetite. The pickles and ice cream of movies and the legendary strange food desires are less common than the need for starchy foods. These now are generally enriched with folic acid, just when your baby needs it the most. Eating a small amount of whatever will stay down is the way to go. And please do not worry; it will not cause a miscarriage if you cannot eat properly.

In the second trimester, salt craving becomes more prominent, as well as the desire for more flavorful foods and larger portions. The caloric demand is increasing as the baby grows, and the salt lets you expand your own blood volume to nourish the baby and give it oxygen. That is why your desire for more food seems to be very common in this part of pregnancy. This is also when you need more water to allow your body to increase the amount of blood in your circulation.

In the third trimester, or late second, the heartburn begins. Your stomach is pushed up by the enlarged uterus and reflux of the stomach contents gets up into your lower esophagus, the tube going from your mouth into your stomach. That causes heartburn. You have to go back to eating small amounts every two hours, as you did in the first trimester to overcome the nausea, and you cannot lie down after eating without serious pain. But this is all normal and not associated with an increased risk of pregnancy loss.

Of course, many pregnant women have a problem of too many nutrients. For macronutrients, too much leads to later problems with trying to take weight off, and sometimes to more obstetrical problems, like gestational diabetes. Excessive micronutrients, like B vitamins and vitamin C, will usually be excreted in your urine and will not accumulate, but excess vitamin A, above 800 IU daily, can have toxic effects, and so can vitamin D in excess of 800 IU per day. You should stay within the UL, as defined by the Institute of Medicine. As I described previously, too much may be related to miscarriage or fetal abnormalities.

Certain foods should be eaten in moderation because of mercury contaminants: specifically, ocean fish that are predators on other fish. Shark, tilefish, king mackerel, tuna, and swordfish should be avoided or limited to one serving per week. Even thorough cooking will not remove the mercury. However, although these compounds may be toxic to fetal growth and development they will seldom cause pregnancy loss, only when present in very high concentrations.

Thorough cooking will remove harmful bacteria, like listeria, which can be a cause of miscarriage. Cooking will prevent toxoplasmosis, transmitted by raw meat or by contact with cat litter from emptying litter boxes during pregnancy. Miscarriage can be caused by such agents, and pregnant women should avoid changing the cat litter. Pregnant women should avoid uncooked meats in general, as well as unpasteurized cheeses and yogurts. All fruits and vegetables should be thoroughly washed with water. Food preparation is as important as what you eat, and you should be careful of which restaurants you dine in as well. Tainted foods such as spinach and peanut butter are surfacing as a public health problem for everyone, not just pregnant women. Most of these foods can make you sick, but not enough to lose a pregnancy. Be careful of imported foods, fast-food restaurants, and street vendors.

Your nutrition is important before, during, and after childbirth, not only for your child, but for yourself. With 60 percent of

Americans overweight, and 30 percent of us obese, we need to pay more attention to what and how much we eat for long-term health and for pregnancy. After staying pregnant to full term, and delivering a healthy baby, losing weight is much easier if you have only gained a normal amount. If you are breast-feeding, it comes off even faster because you need calories to produce the milk. You still need the macro- and micronutrients, but on the same 2,200 calorie pregnancy diet, you will lose weight while giving your baby nature's preferred food, your breast milk.

# three

## WHAT IS A MISCARRIAGE?

~~~~~~~~~~~~~~~~~~~~~~~~~~~~~~~~~~~~~~~~~~

## KATIE

KATIE WAS BROUGHT TO MY OFFICE BY MARY, HER MOM, who had been my patient for 29 years. Mary was still the same thin, tense, blue-eyed, curly-blond-haired woman whom I had treated for infertility years ago. Her daughters Katie, 27, and Ann, 24, were the happy results. But Katie was not happy that day in my office.

Katie and her husband, Tom, a tall, sandy-haired stockbroker, lived in Chappaqua, New York, a Westchester County suburb of green, nicely manicured lawns and quiet streets. But a recent visit to Katie's ob/gyn disturbed her peaceful surroundings with some very unsettling news: three days prior to meeting with me, Katie's gynecologist told her that her first pregnancy—one that she'd been trying to achieve for two long years—was now over.

The mother and daughter sat across the desk from me. They looked like mirror images of each other—both conservatively dressed and looking at me apprehensively. Close to tears, Katie explained that when she visited her doctor in Chappaqua a few days prior, the sonogram showed an empty sac in her womb and no embryo was visible. While modern medical technology is responsible for wonderful things in this world, it also can make pregnancy loss seem worse, which is exactly what Katie had experienced. An ultrasound machine can show you a picture of the embryo and magnifies that quarter inch of embryonic tissue into a much larger and discernible outline on a screen and a baby in your mind. Or, alternatively, not seeing anything at all, as in Katie's case.

"My doctor told me that it was a blighted ovum, whatever that means," Katie said, flailing a hand in the air, her voice shaking as she tried to explain the diagnosis she'd been given. She went on to tell me that her doctor recommended that she have a procedure called a D&C "to get it over with." When she tearfully told her mom about her problem they decided to see me for another opinion. And so, Mary had brought her to my office to see if there was anything to be done for her daughter, a woman whom I'd delivered into the world, and now one with a potentially very real infertility issue of her own.

---

## dilation and curettage (d&c)
A D&C is a procedure in which the cervical passageway is opened (dilation) and the uterine lining is scraped (curettage).

---

## WHAT IS MISCARRIAGE?

Miscarriage—the word conveys so many meanings besides the literal one of loss of a pregnancy. Anyone who has gone through it—whether once or multiple times—knows the sinking, empty sensation it leaves behind; the feelings of failure and guilt; the fear of what comes next. The dark moments of asking yourself, "What did I do? What could I have done?"

The first thing you need to know is this: miscarriages are common, very common. About 25 percent of all pregnancies will miscarry. For those couples in that one-in-four statistic, know that you are not alone. When miscarriage occurs, you will have many questions:

- What is a miscarriage?
- Why did it happen?

- How can I tell if I am going to miscarry?
- How can I prevent a miscarriage?
- Did I do something wrong?
- Is there something wrong with me?
- Is there something wrong with my husband?
- What treatment do I need?

There is medical information that can address the questions you may have in almost every case. Let's start with the language itself. The specific medical terminology for miscarriage in the United States is "spontaneous abortion," which, whether or not you advocate reproductive rights, is a difficult thing for a woman to see in writing on the hospital forms. The word "abortion" is a medical term, though. Miscarriage means the same thing and can be substituted for it in every case. It should be separated from induced abortion or voluntary abortion, which are medical procedures to interrupt pregnancy, not miscarriages.

Before I knew my co-author, Amy had her first miscarriage and saw those words on the forms she needed to fill out at the hospital, and she became confused and upset. She remembers telling the hospital administrator, "But I'm not having an abortion, I was pregnant on purpose..." She was left with a pile of awkward feelings—embarrassed at her mistake; upset because her pregnancy was ending against her will; frustrated at the cool tone of the beleaguered desk clerk; and wishing she could just go home, go to bed, and wake up knowing this had all simply been a nightmare.

There are other terms, too, none of which have a particularly happy ring to them, but being familiar with the lingo does help to lessen the initial shock value of the words alone:

- *Empty sac.* Katie's problem in medical language is called an "empty sac," and used to be called a "blighted ovum." This refers to a pregnancy more than three weeks from ovulation

or five weeks from the last menstrual period with no embryo seen on a sonogram.

- *Missed or delayed abortion.* This refers to absence of fetal
  heart activity in a fetus 6 to 8 weeks from the last menstrual
  period, or at least 6 mm in size on a sonogram. Usually, the
  sonogram in such patients will show the embryonic size as
  less than expected for the date. Often, there is nondescript
  debris or an irregular shape to the sac around the embryo as
  well. Patients with missed abortion frequently have no
  symptoms, or continue to have the normal pregnancy symptoms of nausea, loss of appetite, and fatigue. This can make
  it hard to diagnose if the physician is not sure of the dates
  and the ultrasound is not definitive. Sometimes patients
  with missed abortion will have cramps or bleeding, usually
  around the sixth to eighth week of pregnancy.
- *Threatened abortion.* This is the term for patients with any
  type of vaginal bleeding—from spotting to heavy bleeding—
  in early pregnancy up to 20 weeks, with a living fetus confirmed by sonography. If the blood tests are normal and the
  sonogram is normal, but symptoms occur, the diagnosis is
  usually threatened abortion.
- *Inevitable abortion.* This is the term used when there are
  symptoms of a threatened abortion and the cervix is opening or the bag of waters (the amniotic fluid in which the
  fetus floats) has ruptured before the twentieth week of pregnancy. Steps can be taken to prolong the pregnancy, and
  some doctors are willing to try to improve the outcome and
  prevent the inevitability of the miscarriage.
- *Incomplete abortion.* This means some of the pregnancy tissue has been expelled from the uterus, but some remains inside it. This occurs when the mouth of the womb, called the
  cervix, opens and only part of the afterbirth or placental tissue tears off the wall of the womb (uterus), and only some of
  it passes into the vagina and out of the body.

- *Complete abortion.* This means all of the pregnancy tissue has passed. Both incomplete and complete abortions are associated with vaginal bleeding and cramps resembling severe menstrual cramps. The bleeding can be very heavy at times, so these symptoms should be reported to your doctor and further treatment discussed.

If you experience symptoms described in any of these instances, you should contact your physician.

## WHEN DOES MISCARRIAGE OCCUR?

A miscarriage can occur in the first 13 weeks, or first trimester, of pregnancy, and between 14 and 28 weeks, the second trimester, of pregnancy. Up to 20 weeks or a birth weight of 500 grams (about 1 pound) the medical profession calls this type of pregnancy loss an abortion. However, from 21 to 24 weeks it is also called an abortion by the legal definition in most states. After that, pregnancy loss is usually referred to as a fetal death, since the miscarriage occurs after the time when most fetuses can survive if born alive.

Today, miscarriage is diagnosed early in the large majority of cases. There are many reasons for that. First, about 95 percent of miscarriages occur in the first trimester. Second, we have home pregnancy tests, easily available at any drugstore. Years ago a woman might not have known she was pregnant, and so not have known she'd lost the pregnancy. Today you can tell that you are pregnant as soon as you miss a menstrual period.

Third, because of the ability to do early blood tests and sonograms, many miscarriages are detected before they actually show symptoms. When you have a positive test your doctor will do a more sensitive test to measure the exact amount of pregnancy hormone in your blood, and check to see if it is in the right range for your stage of pregnancy. Your doctor will likely do a sonogram as well to check the appearance and size of the pregnancy and match it with your last menstrual period. The sonogram makes sure that the pregnancy is in the right place, inside the womb and not outside in the oviduct where it will be a problem (this is called "ectopic" pregnancy, and is discussed in detail in Chapter 11). It also makes sure that the pregnancy looks normal based on your last menstrual period.

After that, you will be asked to undergo whatever tests your doctor feels are needed, such as a blood type or hormone levels.

## ARE THERE SYMPTOMS WITH MISCARRIAGE?
There are only three consistent symptoms related to miscarriage:

- pain in the lower abdomen,
- vaginal bleeding with or without passing tissue from the vagina,
- cramps similar to strong menstrual cramps.

---

### abc
An easy mnemonic device to remember the main symptoms of a threatened miscarriage: A for abdominal pain, B for bleeding, and C for cramps.

---

Most of the time, you will not have miscarriage symptoms until 6 to 8 weeks of pregnancy. Even so, you may be experiencing other symptoms—such as menstrual-like cramps, pelvic heaviness, loss of appetite, nausea, and fatigue—which are symptoms that are present in perfectly normal pregnancies. Even bleeding can be normal, as sometimes slight spotting occurs around the time of an expected menstrual period, without any increased risk of miscarriage.

Return of your appetite, changes in breast sensitivity or size,

presence or absence of nipple secretion, urinary or bowel frequency, and mild lower abdominal cramps are not serious indica-
tions of anything and should not send you into a panic. Even
fainting can happen in normal pregnant women (although it certainly seems more common in soap operas and movies!). If there is
severe vaginal bleeding or bleeding into the abdomen from an ectopic pregnancy (Chapter 11), that may be a serious problem and
produce fainting, but fainting in the absence of bleeding is usually
from low blood sugar, a common finding in normal early pregnancies.

If, however, you experience any of the serious ABC symptoms
outlined above—A for abdominal pain, B for bleeding, and C for
cramps—or other symptoms about which you are just uncertain,
always call your doctor. He or she will examine you, get a sonogram, and do whatever blood tests are believed to be necessary
such as for **blood hormone levels**. After a complete evaluation,
the doctor will tell you about your risks, the chance for a miscarriage, and the need for any further testing and treatment. If your
pregnancy hormones are not increasing, and the fetus is not growing or has no heartbeat on serial sonograms, miscarriage is likely.
When your only symptoms are minor and your tests are normal at
8 to 10 weeks from your last menstrual period, it is 95 percent certain that the pregnancy will carry.

## blood hormone levels

When your doctor monitors your pregnancy blood hormone
levels, she is testing for one to three things: chorionic gonadotropin, progesterone, and estradiol. These pregnancy
hormones usually rise throughout the first three months of
pregnancy. When that is not happening, miscarriage is more
likely to occur.

## WHY DID IT HAPPEN?

The most common reason for a miscarriage is some sort of abnormality in the fetus. In fact, it is thought that about 60 to 80 percent of all miscarriages are caused by a genetic abnormality. (See Chapter 18.) However, there are other causes as well. Sometimes an infection in early pregnancy may cause it. (See Chapter 21.) Another cause can be a hormone problem like thyroid disease. (See Chapter 15.) There are medical illnesses besides hormone problems that increase the risk of miscarriage, like severe kidney disease. (See Chapter 14.) Finally, women with obesity or infertility problems have a higher risk for pregnancy loss. Although the American College of Obstetricians and Gynecologists says that half of miscarriages will have no explanation, I believe that a thorough diagnostic evaluation can do better than that.

Only about 10 percent of my patients leave us with no answer to the miscarriage mystery. That means in nine out of ten cases it is possible to diagnose the problem and usually we can do something to prevent your having a miscarriage in a future pregnancy. In spite of the long list of possible causes, sometimes there is no explanation for why it happened. Those patients most likely have undiagnosed genetic problems. (See Chapter 18.) Even so, those problems are probably specific to that pregnancy and not likely to cause another miscarriage. Rarely, there can be a genetic disorder called a translocation that causes recurrent miscarriage, and that is treatable. (See Chapter 4.)

## CAN MISCARRIAGE BE PREVENTED?

If this is your first pregnancy, the best thing you can do is be as healthy as you can be—even before you get pregnant. There is no better way to prepare your body for the work of carrying a baby and childbirth than with good nutrition (see Chapter 2), good health habits, and regular exercise. You should see your doctor for a preconceptional visit to be certain that there are no medical problems (see Chapter 1) and to get a prescription for prenatal vitamins.

Once you are pregnant, be sure to have an early examination and follow-up with your doctor or midwife. You need proper rest and diet, and should reduce stress as well.

After that, opinions vary about drugs and medications, coffee, cosmetics, lifestyle, hair dye, and exercise. I believe in moderation, and will give you my views on all of these things and more later on. (See Chapters 2 and 7.) For women who have medical problems or infertility treatments, close supervision by a doctor is advisable.

When you have had a miscarriage, that supervision is even more important. A detailed medical history and careful diagnostic evaluation is the best way for your doctor to answer the important question of what the chance is of having another pregnancy loss. However, when you have already had one or more miscarriages, it's likely (and understandable) that you might be fearful about it happening again.

First, let me reassure you with this: After one miscarriage the statistics are the same as though you never had miscarried. Only after two in a row do physicians think about an underlying cause; and only after three **recurrent miscarriages** is there a statistical increase in the chance for another—a rise from about 25 percent up to 28 percent, or just a little more than one in four. However, even after three miscarriages in a row there is still a 72 percent likelihood of a term pregnancy and a healthy baby the next time you try.

---

## recurrent miscarriage

The medical term for three miscarriages in a row, the point at which the statistical probability of miscarriage increases from 25 to 28 percent. Some studies suggest a risk of up to 40 percent, but most of the medical information indicates that about 28 percent is correct.

---

Still, the first thing many women ask themselves after a miscarriage is "Did I do something to make this happen?" A miscarriage is almost never related to something you did. There are many myths about what caused a miscarriage, and that it can be brought on by something that you did or something that you failed to do. But these tall tales are just that. (See Chapter 7.)

You also might be asking yourself, "Is there something wrong with me?" or "Is there something wrong with my husband?" Sometimes there is a medical problem or genetic disorder that is undiagnosed or a known condition in need of better treatment. That does not mean that it is your fault or your husband's—neither of you are to be blamed. A miscarriage does not mean that either of you failed in any way.

## WHAT TREATMENT DO I NEED?

When the pregnancy has gone too far to prevent miscarriage and it has progressed past a threatened miscarriage to a missed, inevitable, or incomplete miscarriage there are several alternative treatments:

- *Expectant management.* Here, the patient is likely to pass the pregnancy on her own over days to weeks with cramps and bleeding as part of the process. This is usually painful while the tissue is being expelled from the uterus. A complete miscarriage can be diagnosed afterward by serial ultrasound showing absence of any pregnancy tissue in the uterus, and by measuring the pregnancy hormone and demonstrating that it is at very low levels and declining. It is about 60 percent successful, with complications such as infections, nausea, diarrhea, and hemorrhage occurring in about 5 to 15 percent of patients; about 5 percent of those thought successful later require emergency surgery (usually, a dilation and curettage, or D&C). About 1 in 2,000 turn out to be carrying a **hydatidiform mole**. A D&C, however, needs to be considered by the patient and the doctor to decide if and when it is appropriate.

---

## hydatidiform mole

A precancerous condition of the placenta, which will require a dilation and curettage (D&C) and sometimes a course of chemotherapy. This disease can be diagnosed by the sonogram and is usually detectable by the end of the first trimester at the latest. Sometimes it can be missed until the tissue is examined under the microscope. The hydatidiform mole can be cured almost 100 percent of the time by appropriate treatment if diagnosed early.

---

- *Medical management.* This treatment uses a program of drugs to make the womb contract and empty out its contents. These drugs are called prostaglandins (you may see this referred to as misoprostol, dinoprost, or mifepristone, or occasionally a chemotherapy drug, methotrexate), and they may be given as a vaginal suppository or orally, or both. This treatment is about 70 percent effective. Complications such as infection, bleeding, and the necessity for a blood transfusion occur in about 5 percent of cases, hemorrhage and emergency surgery in about 20 percent of cases, diarrhea in about 30 percent, and nausea and vomiting in about 10 percent. Medical management is most effective in the first eight weeks of pregnancy and becomes less effective the further along the inevitable miscarriage has progressed. If miscarriage is managed expectantly or medically the tissue passed vaginally should be placed in a clean plastic bag, refrigerated (but not frozen), and brought to your doctor as soon as possible.

- *Surgical management.* This is usually done with some form
  of anesthesia and suction curettage. This intervention is a
  dilation and curettage (D&C) using suction to clean out the
  uterus very quickly and with as little trauma as possible. It is
  an outpatient surgery and can be done in the office in many
  cases. It is about 98 percent successful with a complication
  rate of about 3 percent for infection, 6 percent for hemorrhage, and 2 to 3 percent for nausea, vomiting, and diarrhea. There is a small anesthesia risk of less than 1 in 1,000
  for an anesthesia complication and a risk of uterine damage
  or perforation of about 1 in 450. The tissue is available for
  pathologic and genetic study when it is obtained in this way
  and that is very helpful in making a specific diagnosis for
  the cause of the miscarriage.

Surgery may feel like a larger ordeal to tackle, but in the end it
is a brief event and over in minutes. The recovery usually calls for
pain medication for post-op cramping that will occur, and antibiotics to prevent infection. However, most women feel back to
their former physical selves within a day or two.

Most patients cared for by medical management complete the
process in seven days. If non-surgical care is selected, backup with
surgical care available if the miscarriage is incomplete and close
follow-up by your physician is advisable. If you are blood type **Rh**
negative and not Rh sensitized (see Chapter 19), Rh immunoglobulin should be given within three days of initiating any treatment even though the risk of Rh disease is minimal before eight
weeks of pregnancy. If your partner is Rh positive or your partner's blood type is unknown, this is very important. If your partner's
blood type is Rh negative as well as yours then the Rh immunoglobulin is not necessary.

## rh factor

Everyone has a blood type—A, B, AB, or O—which can be positive or negative. Your Rh factor is a marker (antigen) on your red blood cells that is either positive or negative. While most people (85 percent) are Rh positive, a small percentage are Rh negative, depending on ethnicity.

If a miscarriage is threatened the treatment is usually specific when there is a known diagnosis such as luteal phase defect, a lack of hormone being produced by the placenta, or in other cases by your thyroid gland. When there is a known diagnosis in either of the partners or sometimes in both, treatment can be found to prevent this miscarriage or a miscarriage in another pregnancy. (See Chapters 5 and 6.)

When there is no known diagnosis, the treatment is usually non-specific and doctors' opinions will vary. Some doctors recommend bed rest and appropriate stress relief—which, as a person going about the daily business of life, you know is rarely possible. Other doctors believe that nature will take its course and if the pregnancy is meant to be it will succeed no matter what the maternal activity level is. There is constant research looking into the cause of miscarriage and what can be done to correct it and avoid recurrent miscarriage. So much has changed for the better just in the last two decades—in the future you can bet that even better treatments will be devised.

## FROM LOSS TO GAIN

There will always be new treatments, and there will always be hope. With proper medical history, thorough examination, and communication between you and your doctor, there is an excellent chance of having a successful pregnancy. And sometimes, as with Katie, it's just patience and accurate communication. You see, what was originally diagnosed as an empty sac turned out to be an early pregnancy—much earlier than Katie's doctor at home realized because her menstrual pattern was irregular, and knowing that was crucial. When Katie was in my office, she gave me her medical history, which was unremarkable. She had no pain, no vaginal bleeding or discharge, and she remained both nauseated and intermittently hungry—all signs of early pregnancy and not particularly related to miscarriage. What did prove to be of great importance was her menstrual history.

Katie's periods began at age 15, somewhat late. And they were irregular. They often came at five- or six-week intervals, and she was five weeks from her last period with a positive home pregnancy test when she went to see her local doctor. Katie's physical examination revealed a soft, slightly enlarged uterus and all the signs of an early pregnancy. My own sonogram was consistent with the other doctor's findings. But because of Katie's long menstrual cycle, I realized that she could be an irregular and late ovulator— she might be "less pregnant" than her local doctor had calculated.

When I questioned her closely about what her last period was like and when it began, Katie wasn't entirely sure. In fact, she said, it could have been different from the date that she had initially given to her local gynecologist. It was possible that she could be about two weeks earlier in her pregnancy than her previous doctor's estimate. If that was true the empty sac might be normal since it would be too early to actually see the embryo on the sonogram.

I sent her for some blood tests to get a quantitative measurement of her pregnancy hormones: beta HCG, progesterone, and estradiol, and asked her to repeat the tests in two days. The results were normal and went up two days later—a good sign! One week later, and ten days after her first sonogram there was an embryo on the sonogram I performed in my office. One week after that, my repeat sonogram showed a seven-week-old embryo with a strong heartbeat and normal values for all the blood tests at seven weeks.

Thirty-three weeks later, I helped Katie give birth to a beautiful blue-eyed, blond baby girl—just like Mom and Grandma Mary. I delivered a little girl from the little girl I delivered!

# four

## RECURRENT MISCARRIAGE: LIGHTNING STRIKES TWICE (OR MORE)

~~~~~~~~~~~~~~~~~~~~~~~~~~~~~~~~~~~~~~~~~~~~~

## HELEN

"DO YOU THINK I CAN EVER HAVE A BABY?" WAS THE second thing Helen said to me, only after "Hello, Doctor." There was desperation in her voice and that glassy, moist look beginning in her brown eyes as she said those sad words. After four miscarriages, Helen was beginning to wonder if she and her husband, George, would ever be able to have a child.

Helen was about five feet four inches tall and heavyset, her weight not very well hidden by a brown pantsuit that looked slightly too small for her. She looked to be about 200 pounds distributed evenly over her average height. As she sat across from me, she seemed uncomfortable, tugging at her jacket and constantly smoothing the creases in her pants as if the extra weight was something recent in her life. George, on the other hand, was the exact opposite. He was over six feet tall, with blue eyes and light-brown hair, lean, and wearing a charcoal-gray suit with white stripes, a white shirt, and a red and gray striped tie. He spoke quietly to her and said, "Dr. Young has only just met you. Let's give him some more information before we ask questions." With the way he said that, I guessed that George must be a physician himself, and I was right. He specialized in blood diseases, which I saw when I looked over their initial visit chart information. It turned out to be a lucky coincidence, as Helen and George had a few hurdles to overcome before they could realize their dreams of parenthood. George's training tremendously assisted our communication in what turned out to be a very complicated problem.

I began to take the medical history. I addressed my questions to Helen, but George was an active participant in our conversation, too, quickly responding to fill in any gaps that she might have missed after answering. He started us off by telling me that Helen had thalassemia minor, a mild form of hereditary anemia, but that he himself was not a carrier of that trait. Helen told me that she had an underactive thyroid, and George reported that it was under control with her thyroid medication.

When the conversation turned to the topic of Helen's miscarriages, both of their demeanors changed. At first, they easily answered my questions, often finishing each other's sentences and eager to give me as much information as possible. But when we began to discuss Helen's pregnancy loss—two pregnancies at the end of the first trimester and the last two in the second trimester—the couple's sorrow was palpable in their sighs and pockets of silence. This was still a great open wound for them both, and I knew they desperately wanted to make it heal in the only way possible, with a child.

After a few stops and starts, they gave me the whole story: One of the early miscarriages was a trisomy 21, Down syndrome. The others, however, were not found to be abnormal in any way. And the two that occurred in the second trimester had nearly overwhelmed the young couple's marriage. Helen had been treated with ovulation induction for each pregnancy and had taken progesterone in the first 12 weeks for those last two, which ended in the second trimester in spite of treatment. The last fetus was delivered at 20 weeks. Her cervix was found to have opened painlessly when she had a mid-trimester routine ultrasound, something that should not happen before a woman goes into labor. She was hospitalized that day, went into labor that night, and delivered a well-formed, normal-appearing, stillborn female child before her doctor even got to the hospital.

Another clue to Helen's mystery was the information she gave me about her menstrual cycles. They were very irregular and prolonged. In spite of the thyroid medicine, which should have controlled her weight, she kept gaining pounds and losing a lot of her hair, something she complained about bitterly. She said that she noticed that her skin was becoming a problem recently, also, with acne and some stretch marks over her hips from the weight gain.

Her physical examination was revealing in that the findings supported what I began thinking about after taking her history. Even though she was five feet four inches tall, she weighed 194 pounds. Her blood pressure was 140/90, a bit high for her age of 32. She had acne of the face and chest. There was some facial hair on her upper lip, chin, and the sides of her jaw, and there was hair around her nipples and upper thighs. There was a male pattern of pubic hair, as well, diamond shaped instead of the female triangle shape. On pelvic examination, her uterus was normal, but her cervix looked like she had given birth full term. I performed a test for incompetent cervix right then and there. I easily passed a number 8, medium-sized cervical dilator into her uterus, confirming that she had an incompetent cervix because a normal cervix could not be open enough to do that, except in labor.

## OVERCOMING THE PROBLEM

Helen's main diagnosis was "recurrent abortion," meaning repeated miscarriages, but there was more to be said about it with more than one reason for miscarriage seeming very likely. One cause was her underactive thyroid, which needed to be perfectly balanced to help carry a pregnancy because it produces the hormones that control metabolism. If the thyroid is overactive or underactive, infertility or miscarriage may occur, or a woman may have serious complications in pregnancy. (See Chapter 15.) Second, her cervix was incompetent (see Chapter 8) and would require surgery in early pregnancy to correct it. It was possible that her thyroid was causing the weight gain and the hair loss, but not the acne and the male-pattern hair growth. She had too much male hormone in her body, either from her ovaries or from her adrenal glands. That could cause infertility and miscarriage, as well.

I ordered the laboratory tests to evaluate her hormones and advised that no treatment be given until her diagnostic evaluation was completed and, even more important, that she not try to become pregnant again until then.

George had the tests done at his hospital laboratory. They were TSH, free-thyroxine, and total triiodothyronine to evaluate her thyroid status, and estradiol and progesterone to see if she was ovulating on her own. I asked that blood be sent for free and total testosterone, usually present in small amounts, to evaluate for excess male hormone produced by her ovaries. I asked for a morning blood **cortisol** and **dehydroepiandrosterone (DHEA)** for evaluating her adrenal gland, and 24-hour urinary cortisol to evaluate her daily cortisol production. This would help to evaluate how much of the adrenal gland hormone was being produced and whether it was a source of male hormone, as well. Finally, I ordered a blood prolactin level for the possibility of a pituitary gland tumor, which might be inhibiting Helen's ovulation.

## cortisol

A hormone released by the adrenal glands, a key hormone for helping your body react to and handle stress; it aids in the breakdown of food for energy. It is released from the glands into the blood and excreted in the urine.

## dehydroepiandrosterone (dhea)

A male hormone produced by the adrenal glands in men and women. It is usually present in small amounts in women.

The results showed an overproduction of both cortisol and DHEA as the cause of the male hormone effects and ovulation inhibition. Was this because the adrenals had an overgrowth (known as Cushing's syndrome) or was it the pituitary gland overstimulating the adrenals (Cushing's disease)? An imaging study of the head could look at the pituitary gland in the part of the skull behind the eyes called the sella turcica, and that's just what I did next. The results of Helen's CT scan showed an enlarged pituitary gland. Her blood showed a high level of adrenocorticotropic hormone (ACTH), the pituitary hormone that stimulates the adrenal glands. Helen had Cushing's disease. It was one more problem added to all the others, and was caused by a functioning pituitary gland tumor.

Helen underwent surgery to remove the pituitary tumor that was enlarging her pituitary gland, and it was successful. Within three months after her surgery she lost 12 pounds and her acne was gone. So was Cushing's disease. Helen's thyroid was easily balanced to normalcy. At that point, I prescribed **clomiphene,** a drug that would induce ovulation, and told her and George it was okay to try for pregnancy again. After two cycles on the drug, she was again pregnant. I watched her blood levels closely; all of her hormones were normal in the first three months of pregnancy.

---

### clomiphene

A drug to induce the pituitary gland to release follicle-stimulating hormone (FSH), a hormone secreted by the pituitary gland that causes the ovary to ripen eggs to be ovulated.

---

But we weren't home free yet—we still had to contend with Helen's problem of an incompetent cervix. At 14 weeks and 1 day, I performed a **Shirodkar operation** (see Chapter 8), a cervical cerclage procedure, which has been successful in getting to 36 weeks or more for over 90 percent of my patients who have an incompetent cervix. Helen continued to be followed very closely for her hormone status by blood tests, and for fetal growth by sonograms on a monthly basis throughout this pregnancy. I had to maintain everything in balance.

> ### shirodkar operation
> A procedure that corrects a weakened cervix by placing a woven band under the skin of a woman's cervix in order to support and reinforce the cervix. It is usually done no earlier than 12 weeks to make sure that there are no other causes of miscarriage in that pregnancy.

All the while, Helen and George were trying to balance their feelings of caution and optimism—and, for George, there was the added difficulty of balancing his role as a concerned husband and hopeful father with his other urge to remain an objective physician (something that's not entirely easy to do when it's your own family member who is the patient). But as the weeks wore on, the sonograms continued to show a healthy, growing baby and Helen's health remained in good standing—I could see the couple begin to relax a little, and sometimes even lose themselves in the excitement and anticipation of becoming parents.

At 39 weeks and 2 days, Helen went into labor. She was given an epidural anesthesia on arrival at the labor and delivery suite, and then I removed the woven Mersilene band that had been reinforcing her cervix, which went from 1 cm to 5 cm immediately. Five hours later, 8 lb 3 oz Ashley was delivered, crying lustily as she slipped into the world outside her mother's womb. I placed not-so-little Ashley in her mother's arms. Helen's beaming smile and soft "Thank you, Dr. Young" reminded me once again of why I love what I do.

## WHAT IS RECURRENT MISCARRIAGE?

The likelihood of a miscarriage for the average woman of age 18 to 34 is estimated to be 20 percent. For younger and older ages, it is about 25 percent, and 30 to 40 percent at age 40 or older. In reality, though, an additional unknown number of conceptions end in embryonic loss at around the time of expected menses, and go utterly undetected. When a woman has three or more known consecutive miscarriages she is said to have "recurrent abortion," the medical term, and her risk for another miscarriage increases. After two, the increase is minimal, at about 25 percent, but after three it goes up to 28 percent, and even 40 percent in some reports in the medical literature.

## WHAT CAN BE DONE

A great problem that many women face when they experience recurrent miscarriage is that most doctors believe that very few patients need a diagnostic evaluation after one miscarriage. Many do not believe it is clearly warranted until after three. I believe that after two a diagnostic workup should be done, and in some cases if it is a mid-pregnancy loss or a late-fetal loss or a woman over the age of 35, I will perform a full diagnostic evaluation even after one miscarriage.

There are many possible causes for recurrent abortion:

- Genetic
- Hormonal
- Anatomical
- Infectious
- Immunological
- Systemic Diseases
- Blood-Clotting Disorders

Helen had two hormonal causes—her underactive thyroid and her pituitary tumor—and an anatomical cause, her incompetent cervix. Any one of those problems alone would have been enough to cause recurrent miscarriages, and without diagnosis and treatment, there was zero chance of Helen going on to have the baby that she did. The crucial point in her story is the presence of more than one cause. So, if a woman has repeated miscarriages, a thorough medical evaluation is prudent, and all the possibilities must be considered because more than one cause may be involved.

### Genetic

Genetic evaluation of the fetal tissues at the time of miscarriage is often the best way to diagnose the reason for the miscarriage. "Why did I lose this pregnancy?" is a universal question after a spontaneous abortion. If the fetal tissue that is passed or obtained by surgical completion of an incomplete or missed abortion (see Chapter 3) is tested for chromosomal abnormalities, an answer can be given in up to 80 percent of miscarriages. It was a defective pregnancy, and the abnormal chromosomes indicate that it could not survive in such cases. Knowing that it was just a chance happening can be very reassuring. It helps to know that it is not necessarily a sign of a greater problem—and, as most women need to know when they suffer a pregnancy loss, it is not due to anything that you did or didn't do during the pregnancy.

However, in rare instances one or both parents are carriers for an abnormal chromosome arrangement, and both should have their blood tested to find out if this is the case. When one parent is a balanced translocation carrier, that individual has the normal amount of genetic material, but the DNA is arranged differently on the different chromosomes. The result is that some of the embryos will be formed by a sperm or egg with an abnormal chromosome makeup, and inevitably the mother will miscarry that embryo.

If the parent is tested and found to be a translocation carrier, there is a treatment available. It is called preimplantation genetic diagnosis (PGD). A program of in vitro fertilization (IVF) is begun, and multiple eggs are fertilized in the laboratory. Then, several embryos, at three days past fertilization when they consist of only six to eight cells, are selected. One cell, of the six or eight, is removed from the embryo, and the chromosomes are checked. The embryo does not even notice the missing cell, so if it has normal chromosomes, the embryo is transferred to the prepared uterus. A normal baby is the almost certain result if all other things remain normal. The overall success rate is 40 to 50 percent, but varies with the patient's age.

### Hormonal

Hormonal disorders can be another cause of recurrent pregnancy loss. There can be just one hormonal issue involved, like an abnormal thyroid, or several, involving the pituitary gland, the adrenals, parathyroids, or the ovaries. The part of the brain that regulates hormones, called the hypothalamus, may be abnormally functioning, as well.

Once the blood and urine tests show the diagnosis, there is treatment to correct the problem, as in Helen's case. Too little hormone can be replaced, and too much corrected by surgery or drug therapy. Between pregnancies, the patient should have the appropriate thyroid tests, as well as FSH, LH, and prolactin for pituitary hormone assessment, estradiol, progesterone, and free testosterone for ovarian function, and plasma and urinary cortisol and DHEA for adrenal function. These tests should be done at the proper timing in the cycle and for cortisol in the morning and evening to check peak and low levels. Measuring blood levels of free and total calcium will show a normal secretion of parathyroid hormone. When the parathyroid hormone level is too high due to a parathyroid gland overgrowth or tumor, there is an increased risk of miscarriage. Hormonal problems can be very hard to diagnose if not suspected, but easy to diagnose if the right tests are done. And yes, they all can be treated successfully.

## Anatomical

Anatomical causes are sometimes something that you are born with, like a septate uterus, in which the inside of the uterus is divided into two halves, or there can be an acquired abnormality, like intrauterine adhesions from having too many miscarriages and repeated D&Cs. Tests for these can be sonograms, magnetic resonance imaging (MRI), and hysterosalpingograms. Sometimes, minor surgery, like hysteroscopy and laparoscopy, are needed to make the correct diagnosis and treat the problem, as well.

## Infectious

Infections that cause miscarriage are discussed in detail in Chapter 21. While infections, such as listeriosis, can cause recurrent abortion, it is rare that recurrent abortion is caused by infectious agents. Usually, an infection, which is acute, severe, and the first time the patient has been infected, is the reason for miscarriage. Only a few kinds of infections cause recurrent loss. Cultures from the fetal tissues and antibody tests from the mother's blood, as well as specific tests for the DNA of the infecting organism, can lead to an accurate diagnosis and appropriate medication for cure.

## Immunological

Immunological causes, on the other hand, are often responsible for recurrent pregnancy losses. Once the process reaches a level that causes miscarriage, it usually gets worse, causing recurrence, such as Rh allo-immunization, a condition where the fetal cells enter into the mother's bloodstream and cause an immune reaction against the fetus's blood, or the antiphospholipid syndrome, an immune condition that causes a mother's body to react against the fetus. Whenever there is a pattern of repeated losses, the appropriate blood tests must be done. These include blood type and Rh factor, antiphospholipid antibodies, and less common antibodies like anti-P and anti-I, as well as antiplatelet antibodies. Looking for abnormal antibodies is a worthwhile approach to the diagnosis of recurrent abortion.

## Systemic Diseases

The systemic diseases that can cause recurrent miscarriage include systemic lupus, which is an auto-immune disease with adverse maternal effects, as well as the other connective tissue auto-immune diseases that resemble it. Other serious illnesses, such as diabetes, kidney disease, and hemolytic anemias, like sickle-cell anemia, also can be causes of recurrent miscarriage. These illnesses require careful diagnostic evaluation and proper care before, as well as during, pregnancy in order to assure a healthy baby and carry the afflicted mother safely through childbirth.

## Blood-Clotting Disorders

Among the serious illnesses are specific blood-clotting disorders, for example, factor V Leiden defect. This condition is associated with premature separation of the placenta, especially mid-trimester recurrent pregnancy loss. Methylene tetrahydrofolate reductase deficiency (MTHFR) is another serious blood-clotting disorder that in some medical reports is associated with first-trimester pregnancy loss. However, the information is not strong enough to indicate that MTHFR is actually a cause of first-trimester miscarriage. There are others that fall into this same unsubstantiated category, such as prothrombin gene defect, and combinations of the various inherited clotting disorders. These blood-clotting disorders are usually treated by anticoagulation with heparin or with low-molecular-weight heparin to prevent serious maternal blood clots, and incidentally may be beneficial in preventing miscarriage. The risks of miscarriage are outweighed by risks of arterial and venous blood clots, which may endanger a pregnant woman by causing pulmonary embolism (the spread of blood clots to the lungs). That can be life threatening and must be treated aggressively, particularly in pregnancy.

Recurrent miscarriage affects about 5 percent of women, so it is not a common problem. But for those women who make up that 5 percent, it is devastating. The feelings of failure, desperation, anger, loss, and isolation can wreak havoc in a person's life, ruin a marriage, create fissures in family relationships and friendships, and construct a foundation for lifelong misery. But if you have experienced multiple miscarriages, the message I want you to take away from this chapter is this: modern medicine can usually diagnose the problem and, even better, treat it successfully. And, depending on the problem, that treatment is successful in up to four out of five cases. No matter how many pregnancies you have lost, I want you to see that hope remains. Think of Helen and George. Despite her four pregnancy losses and myriad issues that caused them, proper diagnosis and treatment allowed them to become parents. With great communication, we overcame all the problems and defeated the fear that was creeping over them when we first met. They overcame the fear and so can you. Do not give up!

# five

## DIAGNOSTIC EVALUATION FOR MISCARRIAGE: WHAT YOU CAN EXPECT STEP-BY-STEP

~~~~~~~~~~~~~~~~~~~~~~~~~~~~~~~~~~~~~~~~~~~~~~~~~~~~~~~

LOSING A PREGNANCY IS A TERRIBLE BLOW TO A WOMAN who experiences it. To go from the incredible high of learning you are pregnant to the straight-shot down of losing that pregnancy is an emotional plunge that leaves every afflicted woman with deep-seated feelings of doubt, betrayal ("Why did my body fail me?"), anger, and grief. Add to that the questions that clutter up your mind, and you're left in a terrible state. The first question that falls from your mouth is, of course, "How did this happen to me?" Most often, there is no answer given. The patient is told that it is not uncommon, that sometimes these things just happen, and that she and her partner should simply try again. If I were a patient, I think I would find that unsatisfactory. I think some explanation would help me to deal with the sadness and fear of another miscarriage.

Current medical thinking about miscarriage, or "spontaneous abortion" as it is called in medical language, is that the majority of first-trimester losses—up to 80 percent in some reports—occur due to an abnormal fetus. Therefore, the general approach is reassurance and encouragement to try again. My concern with that very objective position is twofold. First, it does not deal with the patient's feelings about the next time, and second, it does not deal with the risk of another "spontaneous abortion" for that woman. Yes, for the healthy 25-year-old with a healthy 28-year-old partner, another miscarriage is unlikely: about one in five. Because so many of my patients are a couple with repeated miscarriages, or 40 years old and have miscarried their first pregnancy, or an infertile couple now finally pregnant, but threatening to miscarry, I have a different perspective.

I believe that patients should be properly prepared for pregnancy (see Chapters 1 and 2) and monitored closely in the first two months of every pregnancy. When there has been a miscarriage, a search for the cause is appropriate, even when it happened in the first pregnancy. For patients with two or more losses, patients over 35, patients with an infertility history, or any risk factors for miscarriage, a diagnostic evaluation when they are not pregnant is a prudent approach.

Of course, every person is different, so there have to be different approaches for each patient. However, general guidelines exist based on the possible causes of miscarriage and how to test for them. As in every other area of medicine, first and foremost is the patient's history. How did the patient experience the problem? What were her symptoms? Are they present now? Next, a physical examination should be performed to look for the clues to diagnosis. The findings on examination are appropriately called "signs." Then come the tests—blood work, and imaging studies such as **sonograms** and **hysterograms,** and finally, if necessary, the invasive procedures, such as, biopsies, **hysteroscopy, dilation and curettage** of the uterus, and **laparoscopic surgery**.

A complete and thorough diagnostic evaluation is advisable, because that is the best way to determine causes and possible treatment, and because more than one cause is frequently found. Let us go through the process step-by-step.

---

## sonogram

A picture made by computer analysis of sound waves reflected off an object, e.g., a baby inside its mother's womb. The process of getting the picture is called sonography, or ultrasonography.

## hysterogram

A picture of the uterus usually made by X-ray or fluoroscopic imaging of the uterus after dye has been injected into it through the cervix. When it includes the oviducts it is called a hysterosalpingogram.

## hysteroscopy

After opening the cervix as is normally done in a D&C, a fiber-optic telescope with channels for inserting tiny instruments is attached to a small TV camera and inserted into the uterus to view the cavity and perform surgery as necessary.

## dilation and curettage (d&c)

A D&C is a procedure in which the cervical passageway is opened (dilation) and the uterine lining is scraped (curettage).

## laparoscopic surgery

Considered a minimally invasive procedure, laparoscopic surgery is performed by making several small incisions in the abdomen, usually one-half to one centimeter in length. An incision is made through the navel (although the incision may also be made just below the navel, I like to make it through the navel so the scar can't be seen). A thin, long tube called a laparoscope is inserted through the incision into the patient. A camera is attached to the outside of the laparoscope, enabling the surgeon to see inside the patient by viewing an image on a TV screen transmitted by the camera. Tiny instruments are then inserted through secondary incisions to perform the surgery.

## MEDICAL HISTORY

A complete detailed medical history and social history are obtained, and the details of any previous pregnancy loss reviewed. Any medical records are analyzed, and if not available, they are requested for later review as soon as they are received from a hospital or doctor's office. Often, the way in which the miscarriage occurred can create a direct pathway for further testing. Pathology reports and chromosome studies on the embryonic tissue passed by the patient during the miscarriage or obtained by D&C may be the source for useful information about causes.

First-trimester miscarriages often have different causes from those in the second trimester. For second-trimester losses, anatomical causes such as **incompetent cervix** and septate uterus become suspects. The **factor V Leiden** mutation clotting disorder, another kind of problem, may first present itself as a second-trimester loss. The next thing we need to check for are known diseases and any family illnesses. These need to be accounted for and stabilized with the patient in very good condition before any pregnancy is undertaken.

## incompetent cervix

In pregnancy, the cervix, which is made up mostly of fibrous tissue, does not open until labor begins and the baby is ready to be born. However, sometimes a cervix may have been weakened due to congenital or other factors, causing it to open long before a fetus is ready to be born and often resulting in miscarriage during the second trimester.

## factor v leiden

This mutation is a genetic condition that predisposes a mother to abnormal clot formation in the blood vessels. When it affects the placenta, it leads to pregnancy loss in some cases.

Finally, we need to know the lifestyle: Is there a history of smoking? Drug use? Medicines or over-the-counter pills? Health foods such as vitamin and mineral pills and nutraceuticals? (See Chapter 2.) People tend to forget the non-prescribed things they take, like an herbal supplement recommended by a friend or family member, or by a "health guru," who often is not even a qualified doctor, nurse, or midwife, let alone an obstetrician/gynecologist. And remember: while some of this history might embarrass you, this is no time to fib to your doctor about how many drinks you normally have or whether or not you smoked or took drugs. Be honest—it's important!

## PHYSICAL EXAMINATION

After the medical history, a full physical examination is needed. It may reveal high blood pressure or an enlarged thyroid gland, for example, both among the many findings for possible conditions that lead to pregnancy loss. The pelvic examination is essential, because it may immediately uncover anatomical causes such as **fibroids** or an incompetent cervix.

> ### fibroids
> A benign tumor of the uterus, which arises from muscle cells
> but looks fibrous when cut open.

## LABORATORY TESTS

Next, the workup will require laboratory tests, usually focused on a
suspected cause derived from the preceding history and examination. The most common are blood hormonal tests, a blood count
and blood type, and blood antibody levels for a variety of conditions such as infections and antiphospholipids for auto-immune
diseases. The common hormonal tests are as follows:

- Thyroid function
- Luteal phase progesterone and estradiol done on days 20 to
  21 of the cycle for assessing ovulation
- Day three follicle-stimulating hormone and estradiol for
  ovarian reserve testing
- Prolactin and testosterone, for an ovulation blocking or
  luteal inhibitory effect, which may create a luteal phase
  defect

Further blood tests may be indicated, as well, including chromosome and metabolic disease screening for both partners. This could,
for example, detect a **balanced chromosome defect** or undetected factor V Leiden mutation in the man or woman. These
blood tests often narrow the search down to one or two possibilities,
but sometimes nothing comes up. In this instance, further testing may be required for less common medical conditions such as
Cushing's syndrome with an overactive adrenal gland, or hyper-
parathyroidism with kidney stones along with fetal loss. Blood
tests and cultures for chronic infection may be done, looking for

**cytomegalovirus antibodies,** or **brucellosis,** as the doctor expands the search.

---

## balanced chromosome defect

An abnormal arrangement of chromosomes in which a missing piece of one is attached to another so that the total material is normal. This is referred to as a process of translocation, because the DNA-carrying segment is now in the wrong place. The person is normal, but the sperm or egg may carry too much or too little genetic material, because a sperm or an egg carries only half the chromosomes. If the half has the extra piece, there is too much; if it carries the chromosome with the missing piece, it is too little.

---

## cytomegalovirus (cmv)

Causes a mild respiratory illness in most patients and is barely noticed, but may infect a fetus when it is the mom's first encounter with the virus and cause miscarriage.

---

## brucellosis

A bacterial infection with the *Brucella* bacteria, which can cause miscarriage.

---

## IMAGING STUDIES

In order to obtain more detailed information, performing certain kinds of imaging studies can often be useful. Ultrasound imaging can evaluate for fibroids and polyps and can often distinguish between a septate and a bicornuate uterus. (See Chapter 10.) A sonohysterogram may also be helpful in this determination. A hystero-salpingogram is also a useful imaging study, which can show the fallopian tubes, intrauterine adhesions, and incompetent cervix. Magnetic resonance imaging can be helpful in assessing uterine anomalies and the location of fibroids, as well. These imaging studies may not be fully relied upon in certain cases such as the septate versus bicornuate uterus, and they do not provide any treatment. For those reasons, more-invasive procedures are often necessary to detect and correct the problem at hand.

## INVASIVE PROCEDURES

Among the most common invasive procedures is an endometrial biopsy for diagnosing, among other things, a luteal phase (see Chapter 17) defect, which is a potential culprit for miscarriage. A small instrument is inserted into the uterus and a tiny bit of the lining (**endometrium**) is removed, usually on day 20 to 25 of the cycle. This can be microscopically "dated" to see if it correlates with the time since ovulation and thus if the uterine lining is well developed enough to support a pregnancy. Hysteroscopy, dilation and curettage (D&C), and laparoscopy are minimally invasive procedures, which not only provide definitive diagnosis, but permit treatment at the same time. They are usually done as outpatient surgery and allow the surgeon to correct intrauterine adhesions and a uterine septum, and remove fibroids and polyps, as well. Recovery is rapid, and pregnancy can usually be attempted in the second or third cycle after the procedure. It is also minimally invasive enough so that Cesarean birth is not likely to be required after having this sort of surgical procedure.

---

### endometrium
The tissue lining the uterus.

---

Knowing that all of these diagnostic and corrective tools are available, it makes it all the more clear that hearing the words "It's nature's way" isn't necessarily the only answer when you've experienced pregnancy loss. After an extensive diagnostic evaluation, about 80 to 90 percent of couples will have a diagnosis—a vital step to getting on track to having a healthy baby. With that said, not every diagnosis can be treated satisfactorily, and for some patients, no diagnosis can be found. No matter how much you want to be treated, you should avoid unproven treatments unless you are part of a medical research project.

Desperation can make a person act not only foolishly, but dangerously. Be careful of pseudoscientific explanations for untested therapies. Ask your doctor to explain a procedure to you before you try it at a private clinic, even if the clinic is on Park Avenue in New York City. Remember this, though: for at least eight of ten patients who have complete testing, an answer can be found, and an appropriate treatment given to help them stay pregnant. Neither age nor heredity nor illness will be a permanent bar to your having your baby. If you are determined, your partner is supportive, and your doctor is resourceful, your problem can be solved. Truly, the answer lies within you.

# six

## NEW TECHNOLOGY FOR THE NEW AGE

~~~~~~~~~~~~~~~~~~~~~~~~~~~~~~~~~~~~~~~~~~

## CONNIE

CONNIE INTRODUCED HERSELF WITH A MILLION-KILOWATT smile. You would never have guessed that she was coming to see me because she was worried about being unable to conceive. She was a beautiful 32-year-old former model with ash-blond hair, green eyes, and pearly skin who dreamed, she told me, of becoming a writer. With such an upbeat attitude and genuine, readily apparent optimism, it seemed that Connie could accomplish whatever she wanted.

Her husband was with her that day in my office. She had met Paul, a tall, handsome, brown-eyed, 41-year-old merger and acquisition lawyer, two years ago. They married six months after that first meeting. "I kept trying to think up things to ask her so she'd talk to me," he said with a laugh. Connie rolled her eyes at her husband, but clearly enjoyed his unabashed re-telling of their courtship and first encounter.

After that, our conversation grew more serious. They had been trying for a baby ever since their honeymoon, Connie explained. She had never been pregnant and was relaxed about it for the first year, figuring that she was young and likely to get pregnant quickly. The past six months had begun to worry her, though, she said, after researching things on the Internet. She was finishing up her MFA in creative writing, and had planned to be pregnant before the degree was granted. It was not happening and now they needed some help. Connie's medical history and Paul's were entirely normal. Both families were well, and her examination, blood tests, and sonogram did not give us an answer. Their further detailed workup was not revealing, and so I performed a hysteroscopy and laparoscopy. The answer was there—she had pelvic **endometriosis**. A thin layer of abnormal tissue was growing on her ovaries and the back of her uterus.

---

### endometriosis

The lining of the womb is growing outside the womb, often on the ovaries, oviducts, and in the spaces between them, the back of the womb, and the intestines. This can interfere with the function of the fallopian tubes and prevent fertilization, leading to infertility.

---

## OVERCOMING THE PROBLEM

I removed the endometriosis with a laser at that same laparoscopy, and two months later Connie was pregnant. I got that radiant smile again, but it vanished eight weeks later when Connie miscarried. The disappointment of trying to get pregnant, trying to discover what had gone wrong, and then believing she was past all the obstacles hit Connie hard. She was very miserable, but Paul was very supportive. He approached it analytically, though, and was comforted by the statistical explanation. Statistics were not much help for Connie, sadly. She needed specific explanations and reassurance about trying again and achieving a successful pregnancy.

After Connie's D&C, the fetus was studied to try to determine the cause of her pregnancy loss. Tests on the tissue showed a normal male, and her hormone tests, taken when she was not pregnant, also were normal. I followed Connie's FSH and estradiol hormone levels into the third cycle after the miscarriage and then her **luteal phase** estradiol and progesterone levels. I performed an endometrial biopsy in the second half of her cycle—called the luteal phase—on day 25, which turned out to provide the answer. The samples showed that the lining of her uterus was three days behind where it should have been. We now had a new diagnosis: a luteal phase defect.

I explained to Connie and Paul that the problem was no longer endometriosis, but instead an inadequate preparation of the lining of the womb to allow for normal implantation and growth of the embryo. The problem was not getting pregnant; it was staying pregnant. They understood and asked for the quickest way to get to their goal, a baby—and maybe, two or three more. I explained the course of action that I believed would be best for Connie. First, we'd induce ovulation with the drug clomiphene; then with **gonadotropin therapy**; and if that was not effective, finally, we'd use **in vitro fertilization (IVF)** to implant Connie with fertilized eggs. And, hopefully, lead her and Paul into parenthood.

### luteal phase
The luteal phase is the 14 days from the time of ovulation to the beginning of menstruation.

### gonadotropin therapy
Injections of a hormone or combination of hormones to stimulate the ovaries to make eggs.

### in vitro fertilization (ivf)
In vitro means "glass" in Latin, so, literally, the procedure means "by fertilization in glass." After using injections to stimulate the ovaries and make many eggs, the eggs are removed

from the ovaries and fertilized with the man's sperm outside
the body in a glass container. The fertilized eggs are examined
under a microscope, and the healthiest looking of these embryos are then introduced into the woman's uterus through a
fine tube placed into her cervix vaginally.

Paul said that he wasn't sure if their health insurance covered
all of the things I described, but that cost was not an issue; efficiency and speed, however, were. He was concerned about his age
at this point of 43, and wanted IVF. So did Connie, now 34, no ifs,
ands, or buts about it.

I started them on our IVF program since the workup showed
that they were excellent candidates for treatment. The first cycle
failed, but the second try resulted in twins. After an amniocentesis
at 16 weeks we knew there was a boy and a girl on the way, and they
were both normal. Connie's cervix began to shorten at 30 weeks of
pregnancy and at 32 weeks I had to limit her to resting at home
with light work only and not going out, to avoid preterm birth.
Then, her vaginal cultures turned up as positive for group B streptococcus. These bacteria are found in the vagina in about 6 percent
of healthy women, and do not usually cause any symptoms. But if a
preterm baby is delivered vaginally, it gets a big dose of the bacteria. Because the baby's immune system is not as well developed as
an adult's, and a preterm baby's immunity is even less developed
than a full-term's, an overwhelming infection can occur, which can
kill or severely disable the newborn. Now Connie was at risk for
preterm birth and a life-threatening infection of the babies if she
did deliver early.

Two weeks later her cervix was even shorter, and I limited her
to bed rest or resting on a couch with breaks for meals and bathroom privileges. Another sonogram then confirmed a **breech** baby
coming first, the boy, and the girl above him, headfirst.

## breech

When the baby is positioned in the mother's womb with the bottom facing toward the vagina, so that it will come out of the mother feet- or behind first.

Both babies were growing nicely and we planned a Cesarean birth at 38 weeks, the equivalent of full term for twins. When the lower baby is a breech presentation, Cesarean delivery is the standard approach for twins (or even with just one breech baby). On the scheduled day, Connie and Paul were very excited, all smiles and anticipation. After an **epidural anesthesia,** I started a dose of an antibiotic, just to be certain that I prevented any infection, although without any labor, the group B streptococcus was not a meaningful risk. The twins would not be exposed to the bacteria because they would be born through Connie's abdomen by Cesarean, never passing through her vagina.

## epidural anesthesia

A method of numbing the pelvic nerves by inserting a catheter via a needle in the space between the vertebrae and spinal cord (called the epidural space). Injection of the anesthetic drug through the catheter permits continuous release of anesthesia.

Then I performed a Cesarean section, but I delivered the higher-up baby, Adrianna, weighing 6 lb and 3 oz, first. Joseph, 6 lb and 9 oz, was delivered by **breech extraction** three minutes later—clearly, Joseph was already a gentleman who knew at birth about ladies first. I was pleased to see that there was no return of endometriosis when I looked at Connie's insides, a bonus besides two healthy babies. And Connie and Paul were just thrilled to be parents at last. Their family was completed with the speed and efficiency that they wanted and the million-kilowatt smile was back on Connie's face, with a pretty close to million-kilowatt smile on Paul's as well.

> ## breech extraction
> A breech baby is delivered feetfirst by a series of obstetrical maneuvers very different from the way a normal headfirst delivery is done.

## NEW TECHNOLOGY AND HOW IT CAN HELP YOU

With the rising frequency of both male and female infertility problems in the United States today, the use of fertility treatments is becoming more widespread. The drugs and technology have improved remarkably over the last three decades. After a detailed evaluation for the cause of infertility, treatment can now be given for many conditions that were hopeless 35 years ago, when there was no in vitro fertilization or the slew of other drugs and techniques that now give hope where before there was none. This is especially true for patients with multiple problems such as Connie. Many wonderful tools are available to physicians today:

- Laser surgery and laparoscopes: These are invaluable in treating endometriosis, tubal disease, and ovarian cysts.
- Drugs for polycystic ovary syndrome: These include insulin releasers like metformin, clomiphene (an estrogen receptor stimulator), and Arimidex (an estrogen synthesis blocker). These drugs have been used to induce ovulation in a variety

of patients, in addition to patients with typical polycystic ovary syndrome.

- Drugs like Dostinex: These can shrink a pituitary gland tumor and block it from producing prolactin, the hormone that inhibits ovulation.
- Gonadotropin therapy: This replaces FSH and LH secretions to ripen eggs through injections. Synthetic human chorionic gonadotropin acts as a luteinizing hormone, releasing the ripened eggs 24 to 72 hours after its injection.
- Progesterone and progestin-acting drugs help a mother-to-be maintain the appropriate amount of progesterone necessary to support early pregnancy and prevent miscarriage, as well as preventing preterm births in high-risk patients.
- Uterine artery embolism treats uterine fibroids.
- Hysteroscopic surgery for various uterine conditions
- New imaging techniques such as MRI and real-time ultrasound

Add to that advances like robotic surgery on the near horizon, and we've got quite an arsenal of weapons to treat myriad infertility issues.

In Connie's case, endometriosis and luteal phase deficiency were the main problems, and Paul's age increased the risk of miscarriage as well. IVF, which is one of the most exciting and effective tools we have today, was their best approach after treating the endometriosis. Other procedures, like GIFT (gamete intrafallopian transfer) and ZIFT (zygote intrafallopian transfer), require the additional high-tech procedures of laparoscopy and are no more effective than standard IVF. They are falling into disuse today.

We've come a long way since Louise Brown was born as the first "test tube baby" in England in 1978, the product of in vitro fertilization (IVF). With IVF, a gonadotropin-releasing agent, like the drug Lupron, is usually given first via injection, and then gonadotropins are injected over several weeks to develop the eggs called follicles within the ovaries. When the time is right, these are harvested by needle aspiration through the vagina under ultrasound guidance and mixed with prepared sperm in a glass dish to allow fertilization. Once fertilized, they begin dividing and are called embryos. After selecting the best embryos through microscopic examination, one to four are inserted into the patient's uterus vaginally through the cervix via a fine plastic tube. Usually, only one or two eggs will take and grow into a fetus. With IVF, we also have the great benefit of preimplantation genetic diagnosis, which allows us to select the healthiest embryos for implanting into the womb.

About one-third of patients have twins, about one in ten have triplets, and a very few have more than three fetuses. But, about one-third of IVF patients have obstetrical complications, such as preterm and Cesarean birth, vaginal bleeding, and miscarriage of one twin or of the entire pregnancy. The more babies being carried, the less likely we can expect them to be carried to full term—in the case of IVF, less is usually more.

In addition, there is a high incidence of so-called chemical pregnancy with IVF, in which the pregnancy test is positive and the menstrual period is missed, and then there is bleeding and a negative test seven to fourteen days later. However, research to date does not indicate a greater risk of abnormal babies with IVF pregnancy. Although there have been some reports that raised this possibility, they did not have definite proof because there are many other factors that could be reasons for an abnormal child in IVF patients. Advanced age, abnormalities in hormone production, and the placental function are a few of these factors.

An enormous amount of research into improving the technology continues. This is likely to improve with time and innovations. Better laparoscopes and hysteroscopes, 3-D, 4-D, and color ultrasound, and newer drugs are being introduced regularly as technology progresses. Studies on embryonic development are identifying how embryos grow into babies and how to help them grow in the womb and prevent miscarriage. Nucleus transfer experiments in animals have allowed one individual's DNA to be transferred into a younger, healthier egg from another individual with the nucleus removed. The result is an embryo from animal A with the DNA from animal B. If this can be successful in humans, a woman in the later part of her childbearing years can have a donor egg with her own DNA carried by herself or by another woman in a surrogate pregnancy. Best of all, learning how an egg becomes an embryo and how the embryo implants itself should help us to prevent miscarriages in the future.

Soon we will have better ways to select the healthiest embryos at IVF, and to ensure that any embryo conceived in the old-fashioned way will have the most favorable environment to grow into a healthy baby.

# seven

## MISCARRIAGE MYTHS

~~~~~~~~~~~~~~~~~~~~~~~~~~~~~~~~~~~~~~~~~~~~~~~~~~~~~~

## JANET

THE YEAR IT TOOK TO GET PREGNANT FELT MORE LIKE A
decade to Janet and her husband, Steve. They started off as many
couples do, simply setting aside their birth control method and
hoping nature would take its logical course. After a few months of
unsuccessful attempts, though, the young couple began to get
more serious in their planning. Janet, a 28-year-old successful
stockbroker, approached her body's temperature spikes and drops
and ovulation days—which she marked with great care on her calendar with a bright purple marker—as conscientiously as she
would her clients' stock portfolios. By the time the twelfth month
rolled around, Janet and Steve were at their wits' end. Why weren't
they getting pregnant? Janet asked me for help.

It turned out that Janet had a luteal phase deficiency (low post-
ovulation progesterone levels), which I diagnosed after a thorough
examination and treated with Clomid, a drug used to correct ovulation disorders such as this. To her and Steve's great relief, she
conceived immediately. In addition to Clomid, I prescribed progesterone vaginal suppositories. I monitored her closely, and her hormone levels increased appropriately in the early phases of the
pregnancy. But even with the knowledge that came with her diagnosis, appropriate treatment, and constant monitoring, Janet was
still anxious about her pregnancy.

I could see this on her face when I performed a sonogram at

eight weeks. It showed a healthy fetus at the appropriate size for its age and with a strong, eager heartbeat. Despite all this, as Janet watched the screen her brow wrinkled and her mouth pursed into a straight line of worry. Following the sonogram, I asked her to sit down in my office and talk with me, knowing she needed some reassurance. As soon as she sat down, she blurted out the thing that was bothering her. "Dr. Young," she said, "I'm terrified I'm going to miscarry."

I encouraged her by reinforcing how normal things looked on the sonogram and through her weekly blood tests. I advised her that now her miscarriage risk was down to about 5 percent. Still, Janet had that look on her face. She squirmed in her chair and twisted her gold filigree wedding band around her finger. Then she revealed the thing that was driving her to distraction.

"Can I ask you a stupid question?"

"Any question you have is fine," I said, "so don't be afraid to ask."

"Okay," she replied. "Here's the thing—can sliced turkey cause a miscarriage?"

"No," I said with a straight face. "It can't."

"How about lunch meats in general? You know, the kind you get from a deli or the supermarket?"

Again I answered no, but I asked her a question in return: "Why would you think that?"

She explained that a friend had told her that bacteria on the blade of a slicing machine could cause a miscarriage. She didn't really believe it, she said, but she had to know for sure. After the difficult year she and Steve had trying to conceive, she didn't want to make a careless mistake and lose the pregnancy for which they'd been so eager.

"I can live without a turkey sandwich for thirty-eight weeks if I have to!" she said.

I assured her this wouldn't be necessary. Turkey, roast beef, bologna, whatever she liked—it wasn't going to hurt her pregnancy. Lunch meats sliced on a delicatessen slicer are not likely to cause a miscarriage, but spoiled meat will make you sick every time, and uncooked meats carry some parasites.

## NO WORRIES

There is a sort of general anxiety that goes along with pregnancy, even in the best-case scenarios. All pregnant women worry about many things, but most especially miscarriage. Oddly enough, you are usually worried more by the misguided advice and incorrect information of well-meaning family and friends than you are by any real dangers to your growing baby. And believe me, I've heard it all:

"Will hanging curtains cause a miscarriage?"
"Do I need to avoid hot baths?"
"I can't dye my hair anymore, can I?"
"Am I allowed to go on an airplane?"

There are a multitude of miscarriage myths about so many things that I think it's best to answer all your questions on this topic now. You may have real, valid concerns about your pregnancy, which I hope are covered in the following chapters. The last thing you need is to worry about issues that are out-and-out myths, or pieces of information with a nugget of truth to them that have grown into a pregnancy-related Grimms' fairy tale. So put up your feet, get all your questions out on the table, and get ready to breathe a little easier.

## FOOD MYTHS

As a general rule of thumb, foods will not cause miscarriage, but certain foods are best avoided or used sparingly to ensure a healthy pregnancy and newborn. I wouldn't be surprised if you'd heard or wondered about Janet's question regarding sliced luncheon meat. It's certainly one of the more common pieces of pregnancy disinformation that makes the rounds—but there's more.

The chance that there is a dangerous miscarriage-causing

bacterial species living on your local deli meat slicer is minimal. Nor is there anything in lunch meats themselves to cause miscarriage. Another common myth is that sushi, sashimi, or other raw fish can cause miscarriage, which is not true (and not all sushi contains fish!). What is true is that raw fish or any uncooked food, including meats, eggs, and vegetables, may contain parasites or bacteria. These organisms can cause infections that might make you sick enough to miscarry, but only *very rarely* would that happen. With that said, I will offer you this piece of practical advice: by thoroughly washing and cooking your food, you can avoid getting sick. This goes for the proper washing of cutting utensils, dishware, spoons, forks, countertops, and your kitchen sink. This is always necessary whether you're pregnant or not, but taking care to follow general rules of cleanliness will go a long way to keeping you and your baby healthy, and you will avoid even a small risk of miscarriage if you eat sushi or lunch meat.

There are certain foods that are not advisable in pregnancy, although they do not usually cause miscarriages. The list includes some popular seafood:

shark
swordfish
king mackerel
tilefish
tuna
Chilean sea bass
orange roughy

You should eat these fish sparingly during pregnancy (e.g., not more than once a week) due to their high levels of mercury. These fish may increase the risk of fetal damage although they would increase miscarriages only if eaten in very large amounts from highly contaminated waters. The mercury contaminants cannot be removed by cooking.

In addition, raw meat, **unpasteurized** cheese, or unpasteurized yogurt are not good choices and should be avoided. But you can have blue cheese, mozzarella, or even the smelly Camembert cheese if that suits you, as long as it says "pasteurized."

---

## unpasteurized

The process called pasteurization, discovered by the French scientist Louis Pasteur, in which bacteria lurking in milk, other liquids, or cheese (prior to becoming a solid) are killed by heating the liquid to boiling temperature for at least 20 minutes. Foods not treated by this process, like milk or yogurt, are unpasteurized.

---

While we're on the subject of unpasteurized products, there are a few myths surrounding milk that could use a little debunking:

- Not drinking enough milk can cause you to be drained of calcium and miscarry. *False.* Extra calcium in your diet is a good idea, but even calcium deficiency is unlikely to cause a miscarriage.
- Skim milk or other low-fat milk products are bad for your baby's growth during pregnancy. *False.* Skim and low-fat milk products contain the same amount of calcium as whole-milk products. Whether it's skim, low-fat, or whole milk, one cup of each contains 30 percent of the FDA's daily recommended amount of calcium.

There are myths about so-called exotic foods as well. For instance, spicy foods, "hot" sauces, herbal teas, and vegetable drinks are common villains in miscarriage myth, but none of these are likely to cause miscarriage. So, if you can't eat a meal without Tabasco sauce, crave extra-spicy biryani, or can't bear the thought of not waking up with your morning cup of chai latte or chamomile tea or V8, never fear. Drink and eat these things if you like, but not in excess.

Speaking of morning beverages, there is some evidence that coffee in excess of two cups per day has an increased rate of pregnancy loss, but this is controversial. Oddly enough, this finding does not appear to be related to the caffeine in the beverage; it is specifically related to coffee, so soft drinks with caffeine are not implicated, including sodas. If you savor a nice, hot cup of coffee each day, please feel free to continue to do so while you are pregnant. If you generally add a sugar substitute to your morning beverage, there is no evidence that these in their varying forms are associated with miscarriage, either, whether it's the stuff in the yellow packet (Splenda made from sucralose), the stuff in the pink packet (Sweet' N Low from saccharine), or the stuff in the blue packet (Equal made from aspartame). You can use these if you like with no known risk of miscarriage.

While we are on the subject of sugar substitutes, I am frequently asked by some of my patients about dieting during pregnancy. Specific weight-loss diets like South Beach or Atkins have not been studied with regard to pregnancy, but my opinion is that it is not the best time for them. You and your growing baby require a well-balanced diet, and this is not the occasion to strike certain foods or food groups from your daily menu. A moderate weight gain based on your body type and pre-pregnancy weight is best.

It is well known that severe malnutrition, such as that seen in starved or anorexic pregnant women, has been associated with increased pregnancy loss. Consequently, if you do currently have an eating disorder and are trying to become pregnant, get treated for it before becoming pregnant. Remember, you must make your doctor aware of your prior battle with a disease such as anorexia nervosa or bulimia when he or she takes your medical history.

## BODY MYTHS

We tend to see both the absence and the excess of every known pregnancy symptom as threatening. Please don't try to interpret those changes because every woman in every pregnancy is different. Pulling sensations in the lower abdomen, mild cramps that come and go, sharp pains in the groin or vaginal areas, and urinary frequency are all viewed inaccurately as indicating a possible miscarriage. In fact, each of these symptoms is seen in normal, healthy pregnancy.

The pulling sensations and sharp pains come from the stretching of the abdominal wall and pelvic attachments to the uterus as it grows. The cramps are mild uterine contractions, present throughout pregnancy as the uterus enlarges. The frequent urination is from pressure of the enlarged uterus on the bladder. All of these are normal findings and not associated with miscarriage. The same is true for the increased fatigue seen often in early pregnancy. Whether you experience it or not, it does not relate to miscarriage in any way.

A woman's body does change rapidly in response to pregnancy. The most noticeable and expected change, of course, is enlargement of the abdomen. However, only after the first few months of pregnancy does the uterus give you a "pregnancy tummy." The uterus rises up out of its usual position and tips forward after the first few months of pregnancy, which is when you begin to show. If you are long-waisted, you might take longer to show your pregnancy. When a pregnant woman doesn't see this pregnancy tummy, it may cause her to worry that she has miscarried. It normally takes about three months for the uterus to grow large enough to rise out of the pelvis and be seen as a bulge.

In some women, the uterus does not rise up in the same way as in others due to its slightly different anatomical position, so that pregnancy tummy may not be noticeable even after three months. It depends on the duration of the pregnancy and the position of the uterus. Some women have a uterus that is tipped over backward, or

**retroverted**. In this instance, it may not outwardly show until much later in pregnancy. Failure of the tummy to "pop out" early in pregnancy does *not* indicate miscarriage, even up to four months of pregnancy.

---

### retroverted uterus
A condition in which a woman's uterus is tipped back toward the spine instead of forward toward the bladder.

---

On the same topic, there is an old myth that miscarriage is more likely to occur when you have a "tipped womb" (a common term for a retroverted uterus). This is completely false. The only thing it does cause is the above-mentioned delay in the appearance of the pregnancy tummy. Other instances of the pregnancy tummy not being apparent in early pregnancy occur in tall women or women who are overweight. So don't fret about it in the first three or four months.

Another common change to the body early in pregnancy occurs in a woman's breasts. In fact, I can often tell when one of my long-standing patients is pregnant just by her breast examination. In pregnancy, breasts normally enlarge, become more sensitive, and many even have some secretion due to the pregnancy hormones. But not noticing these changes does not mean you are destined to miscarry, nor does having these changes and then losing them mean a miscarriage is coming.

However, loss of early signs of pregnancy may be associated with having a miscarriage later on in some patients. If you do have a sequence of the early pregnancy signs, such as immediate breast enlargement, nausea, and frequent urination, then they disappear, along with a change in your subjective feeling of pregnancy, it is entirely reasonable to check with your doctor to be sure everything is normal. Do not feel that you are being silly, paranoid, or a burden to your physician. Call immediately, describe what has happened (or, in this instance, stopped happening), make an appointment if necessary, and have him evaluate you. Usually, a sonogram is able to clarify the situation and reassure you and your doctor about your situation. If there is a problem, proper treatment can often be given when there is an early diagnosis.

Other common early pregnancy symptoms are loss of appetite and nausea. I often hear my patients worrying that a lack of these symptoms indicates that something is wrong, but I assure you as I assure them: the absence of these symptoms is not a sign of impending miscarriage. Neither is increasing nausea and inability to eat. You would be wise to understand that interpreting these symptoms will not help in predicting the risk of miscarriage.

One thing that does affect your potential to miscarry is age—and not just yours. Risk is related to both maternal and paternal age, so it is not only up to the woman. It is a statistical risk; it is not specific to you personally or to a given couple. With that in mind, you should be aware that getting pregnant after age 35 comes with a 25 percent risk of miscarriage. When the woman is 35 plus and the man is over 40, the risk is increased even more, so the myth that it is related only to the woman's age is not correct.

Another scary age-related myth is that at 35 a woman is *most* likely to have miscarriages, and the father's age at conception does not matter. Wrong on both counts! After age 35 your miscarriage risk is only about one in four pregnancies while at age 40 it increases to about one in three pregnancies. However, a 35-year-old woman with a 40-year-old mate has *twice* the risk of miscarriage as one whose mate is under 40. In general, age-related risk for any woman doubles when the man is over 40.

Another miscarriage misunderstanding has to do with bleeding in the first three months of pregnancy (the first trimester). One myth is that it is just your period overlapping with early pregnancy. This is not true. Your period does not come at all during pregnancy; it ceases entirely. Another story is that bleeding can occur during early pregnancy when the fetus attaches itself to the womb (implantation). The only mammal for whom this is normal is monkeys, not women. When it occurs it is a threatened miscarriage. (See Chapter 3.) If you see bleeding, there is nearly a 50 percent chance of losing the pregnancy. However, while this bleeding is not normal, it does not automatically mean the pregnancy is over. It occurs in up to 25 percent of all pregnancies, and with modern medical care at least half do well and carry to full term. Light spotting usually subsides without treatment. However, any bleeding at all should be brought to your doctor's attention for specific evaluation and advice.

## PERSONAL CARE MYTHS

When it comes to personal care and grooming habits, there is a veritable smorgasbord of miscarriage mythology. Right off the bat, let's address the most commonly asked question of this nature: "Can I dye my hair?"

Yes, you can. There is no evidence that dyeing one's hair causes miscarriage or birth defects if you use the usual on-the-market hair dyes. The same goes for permanent waves and straighteners— neither is associated with a significant risk of miscarriage. Neither is waxing, most facial creams, or moisturizers. The one important exception, however, is Retin-A and retinoic acid, especially Accutane. These are associated with birth defects and possible miscarriage. In fact, they are so powerful that they should not be used for *at least one year before* pregnancy. While acne tends to increase during pregnancy, Accutane is completely forbidden no matter how bad it gets.

Also, most cosmetics and lipsticks are not a problem for miscarriage, although those with hormones should be used sparingly. No problem for mouthwash and toothpaste, either. As for dental work, you should feel free to have your teeth cleaned, cavities filled, and X-rays taken of your mouth if needed. These procedures will not cause a miscarriage.

Vaginal creams are products that, despite the rumor mill, are perfectly safe to use when prescribed by your doctor. When applied carefully they will not traumatize the vagina or the cervix (mouth of the womb). The reason that vaginal creams and inserts are sometimes thought to be causes of miscarriage is due to injury caused to the cervix or vagina during application, which can sometimes result in bleeding. However, neither the creams nor inserts themselves cause miscarriage.

The picture is not clear about douching during pregnancy. Most pregnant women have some vaginal discharge. The majority of obstetricians, including myself, advise against douching in pregnancy, because the fluid might enter the cervix if done forcefully. While this is unlikely, I still recommend against it.

Massages, manicures, pedicures, depilatories, and electrolysis are other treatments that I am asked about. They are not associated with miscarriage.

Similarly, I am often asked about the risk of a pregnant woman's miscarrying due to use of hot tubs, hot showers, or tub baths, and steam and sauna baths. Of course, these are known to raise the body temperature and increase the heart rate (pulse) of mother and baby, as well. However, they have not been shown to cause miscarriage. A rapid heartbeat may cause the mother to faint but has not been shown to have any bad effects on the fetus. Nevertheless, I recommend care in the duration and frequency of exposure to steam, sauna, and hot tubs, because of their stressful effects on pregnant women.

Another myth I hear often has to do with tub baths. The pervading story is that water, soaps, or bubble baths will enter the vagina and cause a miscarriage. This is just not so. The walls of the vagina are closed unless something parts them. Remember, the vagina is an organ of your body, not just an opening into it. Even if water or **seminal fluid** from sexual relations did enter the vagina, the mouth of the womb (the cervix) is closed and has a plug of mucus filling it during pregnancy. That is Mother Nature's way of protecting babies while they are in the womb. Unless there is an abnormality like an incompetent or insufficient cervix, which opens prematurely (see Chapter 8), the baby is securely protected within the womb.

> ### seminal fluid
> The ejaculatory fluid that a man expels, during sexual intercourse, which contains sperm.

## INTERCOURSE MYTH

An understandable myth—but one that's still untrue all the same—is that sex can cause a miscarriage. Medical evidence shows a relationship between female climax (orgasm) and uterine contractions, but *not* miscarriage. Semen actually contains substances that cause contractions of the womb (prostaglandins), but even with frequent sexual intercourse and multiple partners, no relationship has been found between sex and miscarriage. There are even some cultures that believe that semen is required to nourish the fetus and sex is necessary in order to feed the fetus directly—but that is also a myth!

There is, however, a known—but as of yet unexplained—relationship to premature birth and pregnancy loss for women who before pregnancy have had multiple sexual partners. Remarkably, the medical evidence does not support a relationship between multiple partners during the pregnancy and pregnancy loss. This means that miscarriage should not be considered as a punishment for infidelity (although, of course, there may be other punishments). There is anecdotal evidence that repeated sexual activity over a 24-hour period is associated with increased uterine activity and possibly premature labor. However, there is no explanation for the finding that engaging in sexual activity with more than two partners before you get pregnant is related to an increased risk of miscarriage or premature births.

## PHYSICAL ACTIVITY MYTHS

Can you still go on long, brisk walks? Is the gym out of the question? What about swimming? Yoga? Jogging? There are many myths related to sports, work, and other general physical activities. Even with the popularity of fitness magazines and literature devoted to fitness during pregnancy, the rumor mill still churns. Can you be physically active during pregnancy?

Among the most common of these myths are the ones that relate to health club activity. Jogging, gym exercises such as NordicTrack or StairMaster, weight lifting, swimming, and stationary bicycling cannot cause miscarriage. Of course, recreational exercise may become more difficult during pregnancy because your heart is working much harder than it normally does. This increased cardiac work that occurs when you are carrying a fetus and its placenta requires a great deal more blood circulation in your body, and your heart has to work just that much harder, speeding up your pulse and increasing your blood pressure.

I would not recommend *excessively* vigorous activity, like engaging in a mini or full marathon or triathlon, or activities like horseback riding, trampoline, or a 15-minute or longer sauna to any pregnant woman no matter how fit she is. We know that they all increase maternal and fetal heartbeat, and that they cause a great deal of fatigue and may cause fainting. We do not know for sure that they are harmless. But we also do not believe that they could cause a miscarriage. It's just very hard to carry on strenuous exercise when you are pregnant, and it does stress your heart.

In general, though, strenuous activity in a normal, healthy woman—such as carrying packages or groceries, picking up toddlers, rushing to and from meetings while carrying a heavy bag, etc.—will not cause her to miscarry. Abusive or traumatic physical activity that would be far beyond normal might be associated with pregnancy loss, but very few women are going to be working on a chain gang or kept as prisoners of war. And even then, women in these extreme examples might deliver prematurely, but only a few of them will miscarry. Interestingly, there is an association with night work and an increased risk of pregnancy loss. So you can work very hard, only not at night! Pregnant women are able to tolerate work at a normal level, without risking miscarriage, when they are healthy.

While the question of to exercise or not is certainly a common one posed by many pregnant women, other physical myths are just as prevalent. For instance, hanging drapes or curtains, pictures, window shades, or any activity that requires raising your arms above your head have been mysteriously implicated as causes of pregnancy loss. There is no basis for these myths whatsoever—feel free to wave your arms in the air like you just don't care. Do the wave at a ballpark—it's perfectly safe. Also, climbing a ladder, stairs, or any ascent, from climbing up a hill to flying in an airplane, have all been falsely accused of causing miscarriages. Regarding that last culprit, patients often ask me about that myth. Does flying in a commercial airplane lower the baby's oxygen level and thus cause a miscarriage? No, it does not. This is simply untrue, as is the myth that traveling by automobile, even over a bumpy road, is dangerous to your unborn child. All of these things are myths. The reasons to abstain from traveling long distances in your last and first trimester are (a) it is advisable to be within close range of your physician in case of early labor, (b) sitting for long periods of time is not only uncomfortable, but is also bad for a pregnant woman's circulation, and (c) if miscarriage were to occur, you'd rather not have this happen on a plane or in a strange place.

Aside from well-meaning friends and family, television goes a long way to perpetuating miscarriage myths, too. How often have we seen a pregnant heroine in a movie or television program lose her pregnancy from a car accident or a tumble down the stairs or a terrible fright? While this may be a useful plotline in a fictitious story, it has absolutely no basis in reality. A sudden fright will not cause you to lose your pregnancy, nor will a fall. And despite what movies will have you believe, falling down a staircase is not likely to cause a miscarriage, either. And as long as we're on the topic, neither will getting angry, getting into an argument, or having someone curse at you. What if your dog or cat, or child if you have one, jumps on your abdomen? It might be uncomfortable, but they will not cause you to miscarry!

But how about an automobile accident? Maybe if you are hit violently in the abdomen, but usually not enough trauma occurs to cause a miscarriage, especially if you are wearing your safety belt properly. This means across your lap, not across your abdomen. So, yes, miscarriage from a serious automobile accident is possible but it is not common. Severe traumatic injury of any kind can cause a miscarriage, but the key word is "severe."

## MYTH BUSTERS

I hope you're breathing a little easier after reading this chapter. As you now know, most of the well-meaning warnings you've received—no matter how logical they might sound—are by and large just pregnancy-loss myths. There are unavoidable things that can happen to you that are associated with a high risk of miscarriage. For the most part these are illnesses. A serious infection left untreated, or any serious disease with a sudden onset of severe symptoms, like lupus, hyperthyroidism, or sickle cell crisis, can cause a pregnancy loss if not treated promptly. If you have strong abdominal pain or are running a high fever over 101°F, consult your doctor promptly. Worsening of a known illness means you should call your doctor—common sense even if you weren't pregnant. If you know you have a major medical condition you should be treated for that and be in the best possible condition from that illness *before* you undertake a pregnancy. Nearly all of these diseases can be treated and pregnancy loss prevented. The rest of this book will cover such conditions and how effective treatment can be.

If there was something I didn't cover that you are wondering about in this chapter, here is my prescription to you: do what my patient Janet did. Ask your doctor, nurse, or midwife, even if you think the question is dumb. And, yes, Janet went full term and had a perfectly normal, beautiful little girl. And she ate lots of turkey sandwiches along the way.

# section two

~~~~~~~~~~~~~~~~~~~~~~~~~~~~~~~~~~~~~~~~~~~~~~~~~~~~~~~~~~~

ANATOMY IS NOT DESTINY

# eight

## CERVICAL INSUFFICIENCY: COMPETENT WOMAN, INCOMPETENT CERVIX

~~~~~~~~~~~~~~~~~~~~~~~~~~~~~~~~~~~~~~~~~~~~~~~

## VANESSA

FROM AN OBSERVER'S POINT OF VIEW, 34-YEAR-OLD Vanessa had it all. Classic Scottish beauty with blue eyes, dark blond hair, and a tall, slim, elegant frame that seemed more suited to a dancer than the journalist she was. She'd fallen in love with Jim, a successful American entrepreneur, whose success afforded them a dream home in Westchester, complete with a picture-perfect golden Labrador retriever. Vanessa's literary career was even beginning to take off with the sale of several of her short stories, a long-held dream of hers that she'd worked hard for and was finally being realized. She had the kind of charmed life that seems to occur only in the movies, played out by good-looking actors on beautiful sets—sometimes, she thought, it was all too good to be true.

Vanessa's story did have a sad twist, though, one that began to eclipse the beauty and the money and the well-earned success. She and Jim wanted to have a child. They tried, unsuccessfully, and each attempt bore the same, heart-wrenching ending: Vanessa was unable to carry a pregnancy past the sixteenth week.

When she was much younger and unmarried, Vanessa had undergone a voluntary abortion in a clinic in her native Scotland. From the dark corners of her mind, it was the past coming back to haunt her and, she thought, perhaps teach her a hard lesson in life.

Of course, it was a notion that Jim and I or anyone close to her would have immediately discounted. We reassured her that the miscarriages had nothing to do with a choice she'd made years ago. But after losing two pregnancies in a row, Vanessa became riddled with self-doubt and the sadness that follows. Maybe, she told me, she'd lost her chance at motherhood.

## OVERCOMING THE PROBLEM

When Vanessa found her way to my office, she was on the fence about attempting to have a child again. Of course, she still wanted to have a baby, but the very real fear of another miscarriage so far along in a pregnancy gave her great pause. She came to me for help in making the decision: was there a real, viable chance that she could have a baby, or should she be happy for the good things already in her life and move on? After taking Vanessa's medical history and examining her, I immediately knew what had caused her previous pregnancy loss—and, more important, that trying again was a viable option.

Vanessa's initial examination showed a one-inch-long tear along most of the left side of her cervix, which most likely resulted from the voluntary abortion long ago. It had healed over time, but because it had never been noticed by another physician, and subsequently repaired, the tear weakened the mouth of the womb and left Vanessa with an **incompetent cervix**. This condition made Vanessa unable to hold a fetus beyond a certain size, which in her case was 16 weeks.

## incompetent cervix

In pregnancy, the cervix, which is made up mostly of fibrous tissue, does not open until labor begins and the baby is ready to be born. However, sometimes a cervix may have been weakened due to congenital or other factors, such as tearing in childbirth or trauma from an abortion, causing it to open long before a fetus is ready to be born and often resulting in miscarriage during the second trimester.

I gave Vanessa a complete diagnostic evaluation in order to rule out any other possible problems. When I was certain that an incompetent cervix was the only issue causing her pregnancy loss, I encouraged Vanessa to attempt pregnancy again. However, I told her, I would need to perform the **Shirodkar operation** at about week 13 or 14 of pregnancy in order to correct the problem.

I performed the operation while she was awake under **epidural anesthesia** by making a small incision at the place where the cervix joins the skin over the bladder inside the vagina. Then, a similar incision is made where the back of the cervix joins the top of the vagina. Next, I placed a woven band of Mersilene underneath the skin through these incisions bringing the ends around the cervix, and tied them tightly to close the cervix. The band was then buried under the skin with stitches. Vanessa tolerated the procedure well, losing about two tablespoons of blood from the operation, a negligible amount.

## epidural anesthesia

A method of numbing the pelvic nerves by inserting a catheter via a needle in the space between the vertebrae and spinal cord (called the epidural space). Injection of the anesthetic drug through the catheter permits continuous release of anesthesia.

Following the surgery, Vanessa remained at New York University Medical Center overnight, but was able to return home the next day. After a week passed, her recovery was progressing well. She'd gotten back to her normal pace at home and involved herself in her writing with renewed inspiration. Still, Vanessa and Jim kept a close eye on the calendar and held their breath. As the sixteenth week uneventfully came and went, Vanessa's pregnancy remained intact. From then on, she would visit my office once a month until the thirty-second week, then every two weeks until the thirty-fifth week. After that, Vanessa came into my office once a week for close monitoring of the pregnancy. In a high-risk case like Vanessa's, regular exams begin earlier than in a normal pregnancy. In addition, today we would do an ultrasound measurement of the cervical length as well as a clinical evaluation of the cervix by pelvic exam.

Her pregnancy progressed normally until about five weeks before her due date. At that point, Vanessa's water broke early, even though she wasn't in labor. I prescribed bed rest in the hospital, keeping Vanessa under close observation. Two weeks later, she went into labor and delivered John, a healthy, normal baby boy, weighing 5 lb 11 oz—and with his mom's beautiful blue eyes to boot.

---

## preterm rupture of the membranes (prom)

Vanessa's water broke early due to **preterm rupture of the membranes,** or PROM (yes, it's a funny acronym for a word that brings up an entirely different experience). This occurs at times in patients when bacteria can ascend into the cervix and reach the membrane around the baby. If the bacteria create a serious infection, the mom may develop a fever and go into premature labor. In Vanessa's case, the large defect in her cervix below the Mersilene band allowed bacteria to enter the cervix and move up to the membranes.

On John's first birthday, I received a small package at my office. It was a busy morning that began with back-to-back surgeries, so the package sat on my desk until late in the day when I finally had a minute to sit down. I took the letter opener that sits on my desk and cut into the tape of the brown parcel. Inside was a note and a small blue velvet box that contained a set of antique silver buttons. They were beautiful, but I had no idea who'd sent them. I opened the note and it all became clear:

> Dear Dr. Young,
> One healthy year later, on the happy event of his first birthday, John wanted to give you a present since you gave us the best one possible.
>
> All the best,
> Vanessa, Jim, and John

To this day, each time I get a new blazer I have those buttons sewn on.

## WHAT CAUSES AN INCOMPETENT CERVIX?

In Vanessa's case, the incompetent cervix was caused by a pregnancy termination she'd undergone years before, which unknowingly caused a tear in her cervix. But there may be other causes for incompetent cervix, such as:

- *Congenital Weakness.* A woman may be born with an incompetent cervix from the very start, caused by a defect in the tissue similar to what causes some people to develop hernias or ruptures. A congenital weakness can also be caused if the woman's own mother took the drug **diethylstilbestrol (DES)** while pregnant. DES is known to cause malformations when a female or male fetus is exposed to the drug by the pregnant mother taking it.

### diethylstilbestrol (des)

Diethylstilbestrol is a synthetic form of estrogen that was used to prevent miscarriage and treat diabetes in the United States between 1938 and 1971. Medical follow-up by Dr. Arthur Herbst of children exposed in the womb found that it sometimes caused vaginal cancer, and often caused abnormalities of the reproductive system and incompetent cervix in female children exposed to it. Exposed boys may also suffer damage to their reproductive system.

- *Cervical Trauma.* Various kinds of trauma to the cervix can cause its incompetence, as well. Surgical procedures such as **cervical conization,** or dilation of the cervix associated with a **dilation and curettage** (**D&C**), can produce an incompetent cervix. Cervical trauma can also be caused from multiple pregnancies, cervical tears that occur during childbirth, and even from forceps used during delivery or strong, rapid labor with delivery of a baby without forceps in under three hours. It may also occur if the patient begins pushing before the cervix is completely dilated.

### cervical conization

Also referred to as a cone biopsy or cold knife cone biopsy, cervical conization is used for diagnosis and/or treatment of precancerous cervical conditions. A cone-shaped piece of the cervix is removed, usually accompanied by a D&C. This can be accomplished by using a scalpel (cold knife), a laser, or a cautery electrode (a LEEP, pronounced like "leap," or LLETZ, pronounced like "let's").

> ## dilation and curettage (d&c)
> A D&C is a procedure in which the cervical passageway is opened (dilation) and the uterine lining is scraped (curettage).

Regardless of how it develops, an incompetent cervix is a condition that usually causes a miscarriage during the second trimester of pregnancy, or very rarely even during the twelfth or thirteenth week. Cervical insuffiency allows it to open *before* labor, from the mild uterine activity normally present. This results in loss of the fetus, like the two miscarriages experienced by Vanessa.

## THE ROLE OF THE CERVIX IN PREGNANCY AND LABOR

It may help you to understand a little more about how the machinery works. The cervix is made up primarily of fibrous tissue, and only about 10 to 20 percent of it is muscle. The uterus, however, is just the opposite: it is made up of about 90 percent muscle. Contractions of this muscular part of the uterus pulling open the cervix is what produces labor pains. These contractions expel the baby by dilating the fibrous cervix and pushing the infant out through it. Most of the pain of labor comes from this dilating of the fibrous cervix.

You may not realize this (or even notice it at first while pregnant), but during the course of a normal pregnancy, there are episodes of mild, short, irregular contractions in the uterus. These contractions will progressively increase in frequency and duration until they finally form an organized pattern of contractions of the uterus. At that point, a woman has gone into actual labor. The job of these contractions is to dilate the cervix (which, as we said earlier, remains closed until labor in normal circumstances).

However, when the cervix is weak, even the relatively mild and infrequent contractions present in early pregnancy may be enough to start the cervix to dilate, even before the twelfth or thirteenth week. In most cases of incompetent cervix, it is only after about that point that the contractions will open up the cervix, causing a miscarriage.

## WHAT CAN BE DONE

Diagnosis, obviously, is the key component to correcting an incompetent cervix. There are some early warning symptoms of miscarriage caused by an incompetent cervix, which may include:

- A persistent heavy bearing-down sensation in the lower abdomen
- Persistent lower-back pain
- Vaginal spotting or slight bleeding
- Leakage of watery fluid from the vagina, or marked increase in vaginal discharge

Unfortunately, none of these symptoms are only specific to cervical incompetence or cervical dilation. They may be found in normal pregnancy in a significant number of patients for whom there is no problem. As for the labor pains, it's unlikely that a woman will realize what these gentle contractions are. As many women will attest, there are so many twinges and relatively minor discomforts during the first few months of pregnancy, that it can be nearly impossible to discern one kind from another. By the time a woman realizes there's something wrong and gets to see her obstetrician, it is likely that the cervix is already dilated about halfway and the membranes around the baby are bulging into the vagina, or they have ruptured and she will be leaking amniotic fluid. At this point, delivery of the fetus usually follows.

Not infrequently, an incompetent-cervix diagnosis is made during pregnancy. A sonogram or a vaginal examination may show a shortening of the cervix, also called a "funneling" of the junction between the cervix and the uterus. The dilation has be-gun but hasn't reached the external cervix. In these instances, a patient is effacing her cervix (meaning the cervix has shortened and is thinning out), but her cervix has opened only a small amount. To save the pregnancy, emergency surgery (cerclage) can be performed using either a Shirodkar or MacDonald **cerclage operation**.

---

## cerclage operation

The two basic cerclage operations are the MacDonald and the Shirodkar, named after the physicians who first described them. During a MacDonald cerclage procedure, a band of strong thread is stitched through the weakened cervix and tightened until the cervix is firmly shut, like a purse string. The thread is generally removed around 37 weeks of pregnancy. The Shirodkar operation uses a wide band under the skin of the cervix to lengthen it and narrow the opening. The doctor can remove the band in labor or at about 37 weeks, as well.

---

If you are pregnant and have a history of recurrent mid-trimester miscarriage, your physician should examine you for an incompetent cervix early and often during the first trimester of pregnancy—but the ideal time for diagnosis is, of course, when you aren't pregnant.

The most common and effective methods of diagnosis are as follows:

- *Hysterosalpingogram.* During this procedure, a dye that can be seen on an X-ray is injected into the cervix, uterus, and fallopian tubes to examine them for abnormal findings. It may be accompanied by some cramping during and briefly after the procedure.

- *Hysteroscopy.* A thin, small telescopic instrument, the hysteroscope is passed through the cervix into the uterus to look for scars or any anatomical defects that could be a specific cause of incompetent cervix.
- *Sonogram*
- *Passage of a number 8 cervical dilator* into the uterus without anesthesia
- *Saline sonohysterogram.* An injection of a salt solution into the uterus while performing sonography to outline the inside of the uterus.

Once a diagnosis of incompetent cervix has been made, the specific treatment is best carried out in the late first trimester or early second trimester, depending on your previous history of miscarriage. In addition to a MacDonald cerclage procedure (which is the most common type performed and is technically easier for the physician to place and remove) and the Shirodkar operation, a few other methods can be used to repair the cervix:

- *Lash operation.* This is performed when a woman is not pregnant, but it can cause cervical scarring, which may prevent conception in the future and, as it stands to reason, is seldom used except with a large cervical tear. The weakened part of the cervix is removed and the tear repaired. In such cases, it is sometimes necessary because the defect in the cervix is too large to place a cerclage above it.
- *Abdominal cerclage.* This requires that the patient undergo an abdominal operation in order to insert the stitches around the cervix. However, an abdominal cerclage is not to be performed unless there are very specific reasons. These might be absence of the cervix (due to it not developing in DES cases, or from it being removed) or a failed vaginal cerclage procedure.

- *Use of rings or balloons.* Various devices have been used to go around the cervix without using surgery, such as rings (pessaries) placed in the vagina in order to hold the cervix intact and keep it from dilating. These have had little success and are rarely used today.
- *Bed rest.* For women who are at the end of the second trimester (at around 24 to 26 weeks), bed rest may be recommended. Between 20 and 24 weeks, cerclage may not be any better than bed rest, but it is often performed urgently when the diagnosis of incompetent cervix is made at this point.

In my experience, though, the best results have occurred with the surgical approach, which usually does not require or result in bed rest for the patient. In particular, I favor the Shirodkar operation, which I used to correct Vanessa's problem. I have found it to be more effective and that it can even be used on patients where a MacDonald cerclage is not possible. Using Shirodkar, 90 percent of my patients have gone to 37 weeks or more when the pregnancy complication is related only to incompetent cervix—and, most important, they take home healthy babies.

# nine

## ASHERMAN SYNDROME: SCARRED AND SCARED

~~~~~~~~~~~~~~~~~~~~~~~~~~~~~~~~~~~~~~~~~~~~~~~~~~~~

### FATAUMA

WHEN FATAUMA AND CAMARA ENTERED MY CONSULTING
room together, she was smiling politely, but Camara was frowning.
At first I thought it was because my nurse mispronounced both of
their names when she introduced them. I would soon learn that his
expression was not a matter of mispronounced words, but from a
bumpy infertility journey that led them to my office.

Camara was part of the delegation from the African country of
Burkina Faso to the United Nations. He was a sociologist, trained
in England, with a master's degree in sociology from Oxford. He
told me that Burkina Faso, which means "land of our fathers," was
once called Upper Volta, a French colony that gained its indepen-
dence in 1958. He had been selected to join his country's delegation to the United Nations by his cousin, the president of Burkina
Faso, the man who gave the country its present name and also
someone whom Camara greatly admired. He told me that the president was modernizing his country and revolutionizing the econ-
omy. As a delegate from his country, Camara was excited and
obviously proud to be part of the reshaping of his country. But at
home, he and Fatauma were at a standstill.

Camara told me that he and Fatauma met in England where
she trained as a midwife, and they had married back home in
Burkina Faso. As Camara began to describe their first pregnancy,

Fatauma stopped smiling. She had not said a word yet, but now she was emboldened to speak, since we were talking about her.

She told me that she had bleeding on and off for three months and then miscarried at four months with a severe hemorrhage that required a D&C to control it. About two months after that, she conceived again but miscarried once more—this time after being pregnant for only eight weeks. She had another D&C following that lost pregnancy.

They went back to England and she conceived soon afterward but again miscarried, again at about eight weeks of pregnancy. She had had cramps and bleeding but her doctors decided that there wasn't enough bleeding to require a D&C. After a harrowing month of on-and-off bleeding, it finally stopped.

Soon afterward Camara was named as the UN delegate and they came to live in New York. Fatauma got a job working at a doctor's office and was eager to try again but knew that she should establish herself with an obstetrician/gynecologist in New York and that she needed to have an evaluation for her recurrent miscarriages. Clearly, there was something wrong and to try again on their own seemed like too much of a risk.

One of her colleagues had given her my name and so, she told me, she had come to see me to get her problem fixed. Fatauma proceeded to give me a detailed and knowledgeable medical history just as her training as a midwife would have allowed her to take from her own patient. One of the clues that she gave me was that her menstruation, although still regular, had become much lighter and that she was bleeding for only one day and spotting for only one more day for the entire menstrual period.

These facts, combined with her miscarriage history and two previous D&Cs, strongly pointed to **Asherman syndrome,** a problem of extensive scar tissue inside the uterus that creates **adhesions,** replacing much of the normal lining. Without enough healthy lining in the uterus a pregnancy cannot develop properly and miscarriage or serious obstetrical problems can occur.

> ## asherman syndrome
> The problem of scar tissue (intrauterine adhesions) inside the uterus as a cause of repeated miscarriages.

> ## adhesions
> Attachment of tissues and adjacent structures to each other by scars.

I gave Fatauma a complete physical examination and blood tests to make sure there weren't other problems in addition to the adhesions I suspected she had inside her uterus, and sent her for an X-ray test called a **hysterosalpingogram** (**HSG**). The HSG confirmed my suspicions: Fatauma had intrauterine adhesions, lots of scar tissue, and not enough lining to support a growing pregnancy. She had Asherman syndrome. Fortunately, I was able to fix it.

> ## hysterosalpingogram
> A radiopaque dye solution is slowly injected into the uterus through a tube placed in the cervix vaginally. X-rays are taken, producing pictures that will outline the inside of the cervix, uterus, and fallopian tubes. They demonstrate that the tubes are not closed off to the uterus or the ovaries and show what the inside of the uterus looks like.

## OVERCOMING THE PROBLEM
Using a surgical procedure called **hysteroscopy,** another type of D&C procedure, I was able to look directly inside her uterus and

see the scar tissue. Passing tiny instruments with a hysteroscope I was able to remove all of the scar tissue. Then I inserted a tiny balloon into her uterus and inflated it in order to keep the walls from sticking to each other and forming new scars from my surgery. Next, I started Fatauma on a treatment of high doses of estrogen, the female hormone that makes the lining of the womb grow into a luxuriant, velvety cushion for an embryo to grow in.

---

## hysteroscopy
After opening the cervix as is normally done in a D&C, a fiber-optic telescope with channels for inserting tiny instruments is attached to a small TV camera and inserted into the uterus to view the cavity and perform surgery as necessary.

---

Six weeks later I induced a menstrual period by progesterone treatment for seven days and removed the balloon. The following month, Fatauma's next menstrual period was restored to what it had been before all her problems began. After three more normal menstrual cycles, she missed her period. Nine months later, Fatauma and Camara celebrated the birth of their first child, a beautiful girl. I delivered their son two years later, and three years after that, Fatauma was again pregnant. But that pregnancy had an unusual complication—not obstetrical, but political.

The government at home had changed and the former president, his relatives, and his associates were in trouble with the regime. Camara was recalled, but he was afraid to go home. He asked for my help and I wrote to his government and to the United Nations asking that he be allowed to stay so that his wife and unborn child could continue under my care because of the high-risk nature of her pregnancy.

Sometimes in life you get lucky. Camara and Fatauma stayed and the UN gave him a staff position. Their third child, another

girl, was born healthy and full term. Since then Camara has be-
come an important member of the permanent staff at the United
Nations. The children are going to school and growing up, and
Fatauma is back working in New York City. Every so often, when
school is out, we all get together for lunch in the city, Fatauma,
Camara, the children, and I.

## WHAT IS ASHERMAN SYNDROME?

The problem of scar tissue inside the uterus is a cause of repeated
miscarriages. It is called intrauterine adhesions, or **Asherman
syndrome** after the doctor who first described it. It is not something that you are born with, although certain abnormalities of the
uterus that are present from fetal life on can produce similar symptoms. (See Chapter 10.)

Repeated miscarriage is a symptom of Asherman syndrome,
specifically if there has been a previous complication like hemorrhage, infection, and the need for a D&C for a woman after childbirth or a miscarriage. Sometimes surgery on the uterus will cause
it. Sometimes the miscarriage is incomplete, and placental tissue
remains inside the uterus and prevents normal healing and the
growth of a new lining (endometrium). Sometimes just an infection inside the uterus (endometritis) or a very thorough D&C to
control severe uterine bleeding will be enough to cause Asherman
syndrome. If too much of the lining is removed, or there is too little
left because of damage from an infection, the syndrome will occur.

When a pregnancy, even a full-term pregnancy, is followed by
infection and/or a D&C, the lining of the uterus may not grow back
fast enough because of low hormone levels. The scar that forms after the infection or the surgery can make the walls of the uterus
stick together. That limits the surface and space inside, so that an
early pregnancy has a hard time finding a nourishing area where it
can attach itself. Without a good start, the embryo cannot grow its
placenta and get enough maternal blood supply to sustain the
pregnancy.

The result is a miscarriage, early or late, depending on how much nourishment is available from the limited lining tissue (endometrium) and blood supply within the uterus. Sometimes the pregnancy continues but the placental attachment is **placenta previa** or **placenta accreta,** two versions of an abnormal attachment of the placenta to the wall of the uterus. Typically, the recurrent miscarriages in patients with Asherman syndrome require more D&Cs, and that only makes the problem worse.

## placenta previa
The placenta, or afterbirth, is coming first, ahead of the baby, and lying over the mouth of the womb. When there are uterine contractions this location of the placenta provides for very poor attachment to the wall of the uterus and the result is bleeding, which is sometimes very heavy.

## placenta accreta
The placenta is attached so deeply in the wall of the uterus that it cannot separate normally, and when the pregnancy is over, attempts to separate the placenta will result in severe hemorrhage, usually requiring hysterectomy to save the life of the woman.

## WHAT CAN BE DONE
As I did for Fatauma, the diagnosis of Asherman syndrome is made from the HSG or from hysteroscopy if a full evaluation, including blood tests, has not revealed any other possible causes for miscarriage. During the hysteroscopy, the adhesions are removed and an intrauterine device such as the balloon I used for Fatauma is put in place to prevent new scar tissue formation. Estrogen is

given in a large dose to stimulate a new lining to grow and cover the denuded areas of the internal surface of the uterus in order to allow for proper healing and to generate a healthy new lining. The balloon can be removed at four to six weeks on estrogen treatment, and sometimes earlier depending on the severity of the scarring.

The uterus is amazing in that any residual normal tissue can be stimulated to grow and cover its entire inside lining when enough estrogen is given. Once there has been proper healing and the lining has grown back, progesterone, the ovulation hormone, is given. This stops the growth and matures the lining so that it is ready to be shed. Then menstruation follows when the progesterone is stopped. That establishes a normal lining to the womb and restores its capacity to maintain pregnancy in 80 percent of cases.

Recognizing and treating Asherman syndrome can change a couple's life when they have been faced with recurrent miscarriage and a pattern of loss, surgery, loss again, and more surgery, repeating itself with deepening hopelessness and despair. Treatment just seems to be useless until the diagnosis is made and understanding awakens hope once again. And yes, treatment will cure Asherman syndrome in four out of five cases at least. If you have had two or more miscarriages and at least one D&C, seeing a doctor for a careful evaluation will often lead to a cure. Case in point: today, Fatauma and Camara have three beautiful, healthy children.

# ten

## THE ABNORMAL UTERUS: SHAPING UP

~~~~~~~~~~~~~~~~~~~~~~~~~~~~~~~~~~~~~~~~~~~~~

## EILEEN

BY THE WAY EILEEN PURPOSEFULLY STRODE HER FIVE foot eight inch frame into my office, I could tell she was not a person who accepted disorganization or nonsense of any kind in her life. In fact, I learned a great deal about Eileen from what she revealed about herself at that first meeting in my office. From the time she was young, she charted her way through life, finding comfort in a well-drawn-out plan and facts and figures that could only add up to their logical sum. And while her job on Wall Street gave her a love for the rush she got when the Dow spiked up or down, she didn't relish those ups and downs in her personal life—least of all, when it came to her fertility. It was something she and her husband, Richard, thought they could plot in the same way they'd strategized perfect financial plans for their future. I also learned about the thing that was keeping her up at night, thinking and wondering in frustration why she could get pregnant—she had been twice—but why both pregnancies ended in miscarriage.

Sitting across from me in my office, Eileen seemed tense. She gazed at me with her intelligent brown eyes, her dark brown hair framing the sharp features of her face. She was just 30 years old, but she was already worried that the potential for pregnancy problems had increased for a woman her age. I reassured her in the way that she was most familiar with—there was no statistical difference from that of a 25-year-old. She also was beginning to wonder if her career was taking a toll.

"I work with income-producing securities," she said. "It's stressful, and I've been doing this for seven years." Her husband, Richard, a tall, heavyset, 36-year-old lawyer for a prestigious international law firm, shook his head up and down in agreement. He was on track to make partner and working crazy hours himself. All of their hard work and long days at the office had seemed fine, but now they were beginning to worry. They had been trying for a baby for the last year of their two-year marriage.

"Do you think stress could be the problem?" asked Eileen. After that, Richard consulted his legal pad and unloaded a battery of questions, making me feel more like I was being deposed for a trial than sitting in my office with a new patient:

"Could the pregnancy loss be caused by dietary issues?"
"Eileen likes to run in the park—should she stop exercising?"
"Can stress become so severe that it causes miscarriage?"
"Could my sperm be abnormal?"
"Does my stress affect Eileen?"
"Could this be caused by some kind of unknown genetic issue that one of us carries?"
"What are the chances of this happening again?"
"How do we make sure it doesn't?"

Despite their business-like demeanor, I knew that they were upset and desperately needed to make sure this would not happen again. Accustomed to setting a goal and then getting it done, they were very clear about why they were in my office: they wanted a baby, and soon. But I knew they would have a tough time tolerating another loss.

I smiled and said, "It'll take at least nine months and you two will have to do most of the work." They laughed and relaxed a little, but I could feel their tension filling the room. I asked them to take a collective deep breath and assured them that I'd answer all their questions, and then explain, after I gathered more information. That way we could get closer to the specific answers to any problems, and I promised to explain everything once I knew the diagnosis.

## OVERCOMING THE PROBLEM

Eileen reported her story to me with the organized, clear demeanor of a well-trained Wall Street analyst. It was a familiar way for her to maintain some semblance of control of an issue that was clearly causing upset in her life. She lost her first pregnancy at about two and a half months, and the second at about three months. Both, she told me, had begun with cramps, abdominal pain, and then bleeding. Both had been completed with a D&C, with normal fetal tissue and placenta in the pathology reports. No other studies had been done.

Fortunately, Eileen's physical examination allowed me to start answering their questions right away. Her uterus was enlarged with an unusual shape, which suggested the cause of her miscarriages. A sonogram showed a fibroid at the top of her uterus, some small fibroids in the wall, and a **uterine septum**. Fibroids alone may be a problem but cause miscarriage only when they shrink the inside of the uterus and compete for the blood supply to the pregnancy. (See Chapter 12.) But a septum will cause miscarriage because it divides the inside cavity of the uterus in half and makes it harder for the pregnancy to establish itself and grow. The combination of fibroids and septum left very little surface to offer a rich-enough blood flow to support the hungry pregnancy.

---

### uterine septum
A growth of tissue down the center of the inside of the uterus that divides it into two separate halves.

---

I explained my findings to Eileen and Richard in detail, and the probability that these issues were the cause of her pregnancy losses. However, I still advised hormonal tests and genetic studies to make completely sure there were no other issues tripping up Eileen's plans of becoming a mother. If those tests proved negative and all evidence pointed to her uterus, then surgery would be the next course of action.

When, indeed, all of Eileen's blood tests proved to be normal, we went on to the planned surgery. I performed laparoscopy and hysteroscopy. These procedures enabled me to correctly diagnose and repair Eileen's abnormal uterus. With laparoscopy I confirmed the diagnosis of fibroids and a septate rather than a **bicornuate uterus,** another type of abnormal uterus. Using laparoscopic instruments and a laser I removed the fibroids. With the hysteroscope I confirmed that the cervix was competent (see Chapter 8) and there were no scars inside the uterus. (See Chapter 9.) The only thing left to deal with was the large septum dividing Eileen's uterus into two small compartments instead of the normal, single, large cavity. Using a **resectoscope** and hysteroscopic instruments, I removed the septum. The result was a normal-looking uterus, normal in size and shape, and, hopefully, in function as well.

---

## bicornuate uterus
Two separated bodies of the uterus, each one-half of a uterus with one tube and one ovary attached to each half.

---

## resectoscope
An instrument that can be passed through a hysteroscope and has an electrical loop, which allows for removal of tissue and coagulation to prevent bleeding at the same time.

I treated Eileen with large doses of estrogen to speed the healing of her uterus and then brought on her period four weeks later
with progesterone pills for seven days. The estrogen stimulates
growth of the lining of the uterus (endometrium), so it rapidly cov-
ers the surgical areas and heals them. After a repeat sonogram
showing all was now normal, Eileen was physically ready to try
again. But then life took a funny twist, as it will sometimes:
Richard's firm told him that he was going to London for two years.
They would have to leave New York and find a new specialist to
pick up in what felt like the middle of their road to parental success.

It was the first time I saw Eileen lose that cool demeanor—she
was beside herself. Between having to quit the job she'd been at for
nearly a decade and find a new one that she liked as much (and
paid as well), and her plans for a baby, she started thinking maybe
they should put off pregnancy until the details of their lives were
settled. Of course, she missed her next period.

Richard had to leave to begin his new job, with no leeway to
stay behind and ask for a later start date. They talked it over, and
decided that Eileen would stay behind for a little while. I advised
her that after four months she could travel and join him in
London. She could start her job search from here and we could
monitor the growth of her baby until she was in the clear to go. I
would follow her closely with blood tests and sonograms and if all
went well for three months, then she could be delivered in London.
I reassured her that the care there was quite good—and I told her
that I had a feeling that this one would be just fine.

After four uneventful months, Eileen flew to London. I
laughed when I heard she delivered exactly on her due date, right
on schedule just the way she liked things to be. It was a healthy 7 lb
boy—they named him Ben. I wondered if it was after the famous
timekeeper on top of Parliament in their new hometown. When
Eileen called me to tell me the happy news, she said that the
British doctor was very impressed at the results of her surgery and

at how well this pregnancy went given all that she had gone through before. "I wasn't surprised, though," she said. "Before I left you told me that you felt this pregnancy was going to be just fine—and I knew you were right."

## WHAT CAUSES AN ABNORMAL UTERUS?

Abnormalities of the uterus are acquired, such as fibroids (see Chapter 12) or abnormalities that you are born with, which are called congenital, like Eileen's problem of a uterine septum. The congenital abnormalities are caused when the uterus fails to develop normally while you are still a fetus—it starts that early in life. So you can go much of your life and have no idea that this problem even exists in your body.

Unfortunately, the causes of congenital uterine abnormalities are still unknown. However, there is one instance that we have pinned down. In the 1950s and 1960s a drug called diethylstilbestrol (DES) was given to pregnant diabetics and women with a history of recurrent miscarriage as a treatment. It later turned out to cause abnormal development of the reproductive system in the fetus of treated women. In a very small number of children vaginal cancer also was found. The drug has not been used in pregnant women for nearly 40 years, but we still see some women with the T-shaped uterus that is often present in the grown children affected by DES exposure in their fetal life. Such women are at risk for recurrent pregnancy loss due to an abnormal uterus. Ironically, recurrent miscarriage was the reason their mothers were usually given the drug. This history is a very good example of why drugs should not be given to pregnant women unless they have been found safe.

There are other congenital abnormalities as well:

- *Bicornuate uterus.* Two separated bodies of the uterus, each one-half of a uterus with one tube and one ovary attached to each half.

- *Unicornuate uterus.* In this case, only one-half of the uterus is present.

There are various partial septum forms, as well. Of these variations the bicornuate, unicornuate, and partial septum tend to be associated with preterm births, and not usually with miscarriage.

## WHAT CAN BE DONE

Late-first-trimester or second-trimester miscarriages are often indicators of an abnormal uterus, and a diagnosis can be suspected if this is the case, just like with Eileen. There are now useful tools to make a correct anatomical diagnosis.

- Sonogram
- Saline infusion sonohysterogram using saline instilled into the uterus and sonography to look at the inside of the uterus
- Hysterosalpingogram
- Three-D sonogram using computer-generated three-dimensional pictures

In addition, laparoscopy and hysteroscopy allow an exact diagnosis and treatment at the same time. Sometimes the problem is more complex, as in Eileen's case where there were fibroids as well as a uterine septum, causing her to miscarry. She had both an acquired and a congenital abnormality. Depending on how complicated the problem is with a uterus, more extensive surgery may be needed. These may include abdominal procedures; for example, for a septate uterus in which one side is completely closed off, or if there is a very large fibroid. For most patients laparoscopy and hysteroscopy will cure the problem and can be done as same-day surgery. In almost all cases of an abnormal septate uterus, minimally invasive surgery will produce maximally satisfying results—a healthy baby.

# eleven

## ECTOPIC PREGNANCY: MISPLACED TRUST

~~~~~~~~~~~~~~~~~~~~~~~~~~~~~~~~~~~~~~~~~~~~~~~~~~~~~~~~~~~~~~~~~

## JOYCE

JOYCE TOLD ME THAT SHE AND SAM HAD IT ALL MAPPED out. In fact, one of the many things the couple found they had in common early in their relationship was their mutual love of coming up with a plan and executing it with the careful precision of a well-choreographed dance. When they decided that the time was right to expand their household from two to more, they began to giddily hunt for a house big enough for the brood they planned to bring into the world.

They had spent their weekends that summer scouring real estate ads, exploring new neighborhoods, and making appointments to see house after house. She said it was a blur of Cape Cods, Victorians, and split-level ranches until early autumn. The hard work paid off and they finally found just the right one, a four-bedroom center-hall Colonial with a big backyard in a good neighborhood with great schools to match—and they now owned it, with a mortgage, of course.

But the surprise that many couples find when they are poised at the door of new parenthood is that a baby isn't the kind of thing that can be scheduled into a PalmPilot. Sometimes, it will remain outside of mapped-out plans indefinitely.

Joyce and Sam settled into their new home that winter and were thrilled when, with the first days of spring, Joyce missed her period. She explained, though, that things did not go according to plan, after all. The day after her visit to the doctor she received a call she hadn't expected: yes, she was pregnant, but the pregnancy was **ectopic**. Joyce and Sam were stunned and then—as when something that seems solid in your life suddenly falls apart—devastated. She had an abdominal surgery to remove the pregnancy from her right fallopian tube.

Within a few months of the surgery, though, Joyce and Sam mustered up their courage, hatched a new plan of action, and decided to try again. They were still a bit shaken from their first experience, but hopeful, she told me. After all, it was just one stroke of bad luck; there was no reason to believe there would be another.

That fall, as the long rays of the summer sun began to creep back and the day's shadows grew longer, Joyce missed her period. Again, she told me that she went straight to her local doctor for a sonogram and a pregnancy test—and once more she and Sam learned Joyce's pregnancy was ectopic. This time, though, it was in her left tube: the "good" one, the one that appeared to be normal at her previous surgery. Now, both of her tubes had been affected.

---

### ectopic pregnancy

When a fertilized egg implants itself outside of the uterine walls, and settles in the fallopian tubes (tubal pregnancy, the most common form of ectopic pregnancy), ovary, abdomen, or cervix, the pregnancy is considered ectopic. The organ where the fetus has implanted itself eventually bursts as the fetus grows, causing severe bleeding, which is potentially life threatening.

---

By then, Joyce and Sam had made some new friends in their neighborhood. As it is with many young couples, it seemed all of them had children or were expecting. Try as they did to distract themselves from the topic of parenthood, Joyce and Sam felt the shadow of it everywhere they went. The emptiness of the extra bedrooms; kids riding in shopping carts in the grocery store; and, of course, the questions from unknowing friends and family members ("When are *you* two going to have kids?"). Despite their fears, Joyce and Sam's desire to become parents still remained strong, and they began to try again six months after the surgery for the second ectopic pregnancy. An entire year went by, and Joyce didn't conceive again. She and Sam came to New York to consult me.

## OVERCOMING THE PROBLEM

When I met Joyce, she was understandably very tense and worried. Her fears were twofold. First, after a year of trying, she was concerned that she wasn't able to conceive; second, both she and Sam were fearful that a third attempt at pregnancy would go south once again. They knew from doing research on the Internet that the odds were a one-in-three risk of experiencing another ectopic pregnancy—which could also be potentially life threatening. The burden of these facts added tremendous strain to the situation. Still, she and Sam held hope. They wanted to be clear on what the risks were, arm themselves with information, and give pregnancy another shot if indeed it was a viable option.

I gave Joyce a physical examination on her first visit to my office in midtown Manhattan, and it proved perfectly normal except for the abdominal scar from her surgery for one of her tubal pregnancies. I followed the initial exam with a complete diagnostic evaluation, focusing on her tubal function and ovulation. The crucial test was a **hysterosalpingogram,** which showed that one of her tubes was blocked at its end, and the other was nearly blocked by scarring around its end. She probably had a mild infection of her tubes years before her first pregnancy. Frequently, this type of infection is unnoticed or causes minor symptoms for only a few days and then it subsides without treatment. However, the damage has been done.

I performed laparoscopic surgery to correct her tubal disease and I was able to open both tubes. Six days later, I did a post-operative hysterosalpingogram to see the results of the laparoscopy. Now I could see that both tubes were wide open.

---

## hysterosalpingogram

A radiopaque dye solution is slowly injected into the uterus through a tube placed in the cervix vaginally. X-rays are taken, producing pictures that will outline the inside of the cervix, uterus, and fallopian tubes. They demonstrate that the tubes are not closed off to the uterus or the ovaries and show what the inside of the uterus looks like.

---

With the problem corrected, I gave Joyce and Sam the green light to try again, but warned them that there was still a 20 percent risk of another ectopic pregnancy. I made it clear that they should get in touch with me as soon as Joyce thought she might be pregnant. To their great relief, Joyce conceived within a few months. From that point forward, I followed the pregnancy's progress very closely, using serial sonograms and **blood hormone tests** beta HCG, estradiol, and progesterone every three days to track the first three critical months of the pregnancy. Also, sonograms confirmed that the pregnancy was in the right place. Month after month went by and the pregnancy progressed normally within the uterus, where it belonged.

During a happily uneventful delivery, Joyce and Sam's beautiful daughter, Abigail, was delivered at full term—7 lb 4 oz of joyfully kicking, squealing, and squirming baby.

## WHAT CAUSES THE PROBLEM?

When a pregnancy is ectopic, that means it occurs in a place other than where it's supposed to be (e.g., the uterus). Ectopic pregnancy can occur within the fallopian tube, the ovaries, the cervix, and even within the abdominal cavity. However, the most common site is within the fallopian tube, as we saw with Joyce. The fallopian tube is the passageway that the egg follows from the ovary into the uterus. In a normal pregnancy, the fertilized egg finds its way through the fallopian tube and attaches itself in the uterus. But in a tubal pregnancy, the egg becomes stuck in the fallopian tube. In Joyce's case, there was blockage and scarring in her fallopian tubes. That's why the fertilized eggs from her first two pregnancies couldn't make the journey into the uterus.

What causes pregnancy problems in the fallopian tubes? The most common causes are related to factors like:

- **Pelvic inflammatory disease** (**PID**) involving the fallopian tubes, like sexually transmitted infections (STIs)
- Anatomical abnormalities such as **DES** exposure, congenital narrowing of the tube, or other tubal malformations
- Hormonal disturbances, like low estrogen levels
- Delayed ovulation resulting in tubal dysfunction
- Intrauterine devices, which only prevent uterine pregnancy, not tubal pregnancy
- Transport of the egg across to the tube on the opposite side. The egg is not picked up by the tube next to the ovary it came from; instead it drifts to the other side and is picked up by the opposite tube.
- In vitro fertilization

## pelvic inflammatory disease (pid)

PID is an infection often caused by sexually transmitted organisms (most often chlamydia or gonorrhea), affecting a woman's reproductive organs. Symptoms of PID include fever, painful urination, painful intercourse, irregular menstrual bleeding, and an odorous vaginal discharge. Sometimes symptoms are mild and may go away quickly, but the damage to the tubes may still occur. Rarely, a sore throat or respiratory infection may enter the bloodstream and land in the tubes, causing PID from a non–sexually transmitted source.

## diethylstilbestrol (des)

Diethylstilbestrol is a synthetic form of estrogen that was used to prevent miscarriage and treat diabetes in the U.S. between 1938 and 1971. Medical follow-up by Dr. Arthur Herbst of children exposed in the womb found that it sometimes caused vaginal cancer, and often caused abnormalities of the reproductive system and incompetent cervix in female children exposed to it. Exposed boys may also suffer damage to their reproductive system.

About 1 in 60 pregnancies in the United States is ectopic, and the rate is increasing every year. Tubal pregnancy in particular is becoming more and more common. The occurrence has increased four times over the last 25 years at a rate of about 10 percent per year. And, unfortunately, it shows no signs of slowing down. The most likely explanation for the increase is widespread sexually transmitted disease, all too frequently undiagnosed and untreated. The risk of dying from a tubal pregnancy is about 5 in 10,000. It is the most common cause of maternal death during the first 20 weeks of pregnancy, and 100 percent of the babies die. Also, unlike other pregnancy issues that are affected by age or even race, tubal pregnancy is indiscriminate. It can affect a woman of any age or race.

Most ectopic pregnancies occur in the fallopian tube because the tube is very narrow. Its wall is also thin and easily damaged both inside and out. Each of these factors means that, after an egg has been fertilized within a damaged tube and begins its journey through it, the egg's path may well be blocked. When the tube is not damaged but its normal motion is disturbed, the egg may be delayed in its passage through the tube. This can occur due to abnormal hormones or from an intrauterine device. With in vitro fertilization, it is thought that the embryo fails to attach to the wall of the uterus and somehow finds its way backward up into the oviduct, possibly due to the way the catheter is placed into the uterus during embryo transfer. In other ectopic pregnancies, the egg is fertilized *outside* the tube also and may attach itself to the ovary or to other abdominal organs, the upshot being an ovarian pregnancy or, even more rare, an abdominal pregnancy.

When the ectopic pregnancy occurs at the end of the tube near the ovary, it's possible that it may go away by itself, breaking off and passing out the open end of the tube (this is also called a tubal abortion). However, it may also begin to grow within the wall of the tube until the thin wall bursts and hemorrhage occurs. When the ectopic pregnancy is in the part of the tube that runs through the wall of the uterus, it is called an **interstitial pregnancy**. This type may grow to a substantial size before it ruptures, which often occurs in about the fourth month of pregnancy. This is later than most tubal pregnancies, therefore bigger. The rupture is usually accompanied by rapid, severe abdominal hemorrhage. This bleeding can very quickly be fatal.

---

### interstitial pregnancy

An ectopic pregnancy that develops in the uterine, or interstitial, section of the fallopian tube.

---

Most cases of tubal pregnancy will rupture earlier, usually within the first three months. If this is the case, the rupture can be very dangerous to the pregnant woman's health, causing major bleeding into the abdomen. If the hemorrhage is severe enough, the patient may die.

Ovarian pregnancy is a lot like a tubal pregnancy. The abdominal pregnancy, however, may go on up to the third trimester, although this happens very rarely. There are even cases where the pregnancy went full term. As you might imagine, the latter example is an exception to the exception—it rarely happens. Unfortunately, the reality is that most ectopic pregnancies end in the loss of the fetus.

Although rare, the last type of ectopic pregnancy that you should be aware of is a cervical pregnancy. In this case, the ovum travels through the uterus and attaches in the cervix, poised on the verge of miscarrying. Bleeding begins within the first two weeks of a cervical ectopic pregnancy, and becomes increasingly heavier as the pregnancy continues (usually until about the eighth week). Once diagnosed, this type of ectopic pregnancy is often treated by injection of a toxic agent into the pregnancy to destroy the placenta, in conjunction with a second drug sometimes given to the pregnant woman. If the drugs are not sufficient to end the pregnancy and surgery is required, a substantial amount of bleeding is to be expected and, sometimes, a hysterectomy may even be necessary. The bleeding comes from the large blood vessels that have grown to feed the pregnancy. Controlling the bleeding from these vessels in the cervix is very difficult, especially if a D&C is attempted.

## WHAT CAN BE DONE

Joyce was very fortunate. Following a proper and thorough diagnosis, it was clear to me that I could fix her problem with laparoscopic surgery. Even though the solution is not always as readily handy as this, the overwhelming majority of ectopic pregnancies are tubal and can be diagnosed in a few different ways. First, the medical history may give us some clues:

- The patient has a pre-existing pelvic infection or infertility.
- The patient had or presently has an IUD.

- The patient suffers from **endometriosis**.
- The patient has had pelvic or abdominal surgery that has left scarring on the fallopian tubes.
- The patient experiences a delay in her menstrual period followed by spotting, or delayed or abnormal menstruation as well as abdominal pain and a positive pregnancy test.

---

### endometriosis
The lining of the womb is growing outside the womb, often on the ovaries, oviducts, and in the spaces between them, the back of the womb, and the intestines. This can interfere with the function of the fallopian tubes and prevent fertilization, leading to infertility.

---

The following symptoms are also possible telltale signs of an ectopic pregnancy:

abdominal pain
shoulder or neck pain
dizziness
weakness
fainting
very rapid heartbeat
vaginal bleeding

The problem, of course (which is the problem with most instances of miscarriage), is that many of the symptoms of an ectopic pregnancy are just like those of a normal pregnancy or a threatened miscarriage, and are easily confused with those conditions. But following a careful look at the patient's history, a doctor who suspects a patient might be experiencing ectopic pregnancy can diagnose it with the following methods:

- Physical examination
- Ultrasound showing pregnancy outside the uterus (a vaginal ultrasound probe is especially useful to detect ectopic pregnancy)
- Blood hormone tests, specifically for quantitative beta **HCG,** progesterone, and estradiol
- Complete blood count

---

## hcg

Human chorionic gonodotropin (HCG) is a hormone produced by the growing placenta.

---

Sometimes, it can be difficult to come up with a diagnosis right away, so the tests are usually repeated in two to seven days until the problem reveals itself. When it does, laparoscopy is performed for diagnosis and treatment, as in Joyce's case, and sometimes an abdominal operation is necessary as part of the treatment, as well, if there already is a hemorrhage. During laparoscopy, a telescope-like tube with a TV camera attachment is inserted through a small incision to the patient's abdominal wall, allowing the surgeon to look at the pelvic organs.

During treatment, special instruments such as a laser, or a fine needle cautery, are used to remove the ectopic pregnancy and, just like with Joyce's treatment, the patient's tube usually heals. Many women can go home the day after or even the same day. The healing time required is also very minimal (although sometimes excessive bleeding caused by the ectopic pregnancy will necessitate an abdominal incision in order to control the bleeding and remove the leftover pregnancy tissue). The good news is that the tube is rarely damaged to the point where it can't be saved and needs to be removed.

There are other alternatives to the surgical approach if an ectopic pregnancy is diagnosed very early and has not grown to a substantial size. This is why it is *imperative* that your doctor is up to speed on your medical history—if you leave something out, it may cause him or her to misdiagnose you from the outset, causing you to lose precious time and, potentially, put your fertility and even your life at risk. With early diagnosis, the mother may be given an injection or oral dose of a drug called methotrexate, which will destroy the pregnancy tissue, allowing the tube to absorb it and heal spontaneously. There are also certain patients in whom the ectopic pregnancy ends in the fallopian tube without any distress to the mother, and is absorbed without leaving any residual damage.

Non-surgical methods might be an easier way of getting past an ectopic pregnancy, but there are risks of toxic effects from the drug. While these methods have been shown to leave a woman with the same degree of fertility as surgery, about 20 to 30 percent of non-surgical methods will end up resulting in an emergency surgery anyway. Laparoscopy is the preferred treatment for ectopic pregnancy when there is a pregnancy past six weeks or bleeding. The long-term prognosis using either treatment is approximately an 80 percent pregnancy rate, with 70 percent of those being normal (10 percent are ectopic, which works out to be between a 9 and 19 percent recurrence rate following one ectopic pregnancy; and between 10 and 40 percent following a second one).

Even if you're not handy with a calculator, you can see that all this shakes out to be about a 20 percent rate of infertility after one ectopic pregnancy.

But let's look to Joyce for a moment. Despite having miscarriages due to two ectopic pregnancies, she went on to have a normal pregnancy and normal childbirth. Because of the clear line of communication between patient and doctor, and the advances in diagnosis and treatment, I was able to properly care for her. After laparoscopic surgery, the path was cleared—and now Joyce and Sam have Abigail. Treatment like this, as well as the enormous potential of in vitro fertilization, shift the outlook for a woman who has endured tubal pregnancy from a mere roll of the dice to a child well within her grasp. Even if both tubes are gone, the power of technology with in vitro fertilization offers about a 60 percent likelihood for a normal pregnancy. With medical or surgical treatment of an ectopic tubal pregnancy, conserving the tubes gives you about an 80 percent chance of bringing home your baby. What once was a life-threatening disease usually causing sterility is today cured in the majority of women.

# twelve

## FIBROIDS: UNWANTED GUESTS

~~~~~~~~~~~~~~~~~~~~~~~~~~~~~~~~~~~~~~~~~~~~~~~~~~~~~~~~~

## SHANITRA

SHANITRA CAME TO SEE ME BECAUSE SHE HAD LOST three pregnancies within two years. She explained that after each loss, insult was added to painful injury when her former physician told her she couldn't see any reason why Shanitra was miscarrying; there was nothing wrong. All around her, it seemed to her, there were pregnant women. On the sidewalks, in the supermarket, at the movie-rental shop. Everywhere she went, there was another swelled belly on another lucky woman, she said, almost angry.

Her friends were all having babies, she said, a trace of jealousy in her tone. Even her co-workers at the bank were making happy announcements and going on maternity leave. Invitations to baby showers became more common than junk mail, she lamented. Even worse, from after her first pregnancy and subsequent miscarriages, her health-insurance provider started sending mommy-and-baby-wellness literature. Shanitra would take this out of her mailbox and quickly toss it in the recycle bin. Babies and information about them and how wonderful it was to be a mother seemed to be unavoidable. How wonderful it was to be a mother seemed to apply to everyone but her, she told me.

Shanitra had stopped taking her birth control pills two years ago after she and her husband, Michael, were married. Michael worked at my hospital as a records coordinator, and between them (she was an employee at a major New York bank) they had very good health insurance, so Shanitra decided she needed to see another doctor. Michael inquired among the hospital personnel he knew, and that's how Shanitra came to see me.

She had a totally normal medical history. Shanitra felt that her periods were normal if somewhat heavier in the past two years when she stopped taking the oral contraceptive pill. Starting from the age of 18, she'd been on the pill steadily for nine years and had been accustomed to a light flow, which she'd always chalked up to a side effect of her birth control. She was almost 28 years old now, she said wistfully.

"I used to hear women talking about how badly they wanted a child, and I thought they were weird," she told me in my office that day. "But now...I feel like I *need* a child. That sounds crazy, right?"

Of course, I told her, it didn't. I'd met thousands of patients over the years whose reactions to parenthood ran the gamut from terrified to yearning to ambivalence to a calling. There is no "right" reaction to becoming a mom or dealing with infertility issues. It certainly is a difficult plight in which some couples are surprised to find themselves, and they react in different ways.

And so, we started with a full medical workup. Her physical examination turned up just one abnormal finding. Her uterus was enlarged to almost the size of a ten-weeks pregnancy. It felt like a **fibroid,** and a sonogram showed a fibroid tumor in the front wall of her uterus. A **sonohysterogram** confirmed that the fibroid bulged into the cavity of the uterus. Only about one-fourth of the fibroid pushed into the uterine cavity, and the remaining three-fourths was occupying the wall of the uterus. The fibroid tumor was actually larger than the uterus and compressed it, completely taking up the top and front walls of Shanitra's womb. A pregnancy test was negative, as were all her hormone tests. Her genetics studies were normal.

## fibroid
A benign tumor of the uterus, which arises from muscle cells but looks fibrous when cut open.

## sonohysterogram
A sterile solution is instilled vaginally through the cervix into the uterus and ultrasound pictures are taken to outline the uterus and the inside cavity of the uterus.

Taking up all this space in her womb not only left no room for a fetus to grow, it also directed most of the blood supply to the tumor, leaving very little to support a pregnancy. Fortunately, Shanitra had no problem getting pregnant because she and Michael were normal in every way—no hormone problems, no genetic problems, and no other major or even minor medical issues. The exception was just this: one big fibroid.

## OVERCOMING THE PROBLEM
For Shanitra, a pregnancy could get started, but lacking enough blood and nutritional lining to support it, the pregnancy could get just so far. In her case, that translated into eight to ten weeks of pregnancy, and then an inevitable miscarriage. I explained this to Shanitra and Michael, as well as to Shanitra's mom, Etheline, who was invited by her daughter to join us because Etheline was a licensed practical nurse—as well as a concerned mom who was worried about her daughter.

I explained fibroid tumors to the family and recommended an abdominal **myomectomy** for Shanitra since vaginal surgery and laparoscopic surgery were not likely to be successful in her case.

The other procedures could be used in specific instances when the tumor was smaller, or when more than two-thirds of it was within the uterine cavity. But this one was large and nearly went through the full thickness of the wall of the womb. I drew pictures outlining the location of the fibroid so they could visualize the problem, and discussed which kind of a surgical procedure would be necessary to remove it. Among other things, I also explained to them that with any myomectomy, there is a risk of post-surgical scarring that can prevent a future pregnancy. However, I emphasized that the percentage for this is very low—only 10 percent of women will develop this type of scar tissue involving the uterine lining or around the oviducts.

> ## myomectomy
> An operation to remove a fibroid or fibroids.

After hearing my recommendation and all the information surrounding it, they had many questions. "How long is the hospital stay? Is it painful? How long do I have to wait to get pregnant after the operation?" After I answered their questions, the family was still undecided and needed to take some time to think about how to proceed. They were not worried about the risks of surgery at all, they said. Just had to sort out all the information, they told me. I advised Shanitra and Michael to use condom contraception while they thought it over, as I did not want them to go through another miscarriage. Shanitra asked me if she could just go back on birth control pills. As it so happens, oral contraceptive pills were likely part of the problem to begin with for Shanitra because they can stimulate fibroids to grow. Fibroids have receptors for estrogen and progesterone, the ingredients in birth control pills. That could only make the situation worse. After they said good-bye, they were talking among themselves as they left my consulting room and appeared to be agreeing on something.

The next morning Shanitra called to schedule her surgery, and I scheduled her myomectomy for two weeks later. I performed a "bikini incision," a cut at the pubic hairline that leaves a nearly unnoticeable scar, and removed the fibroid without cutting into the lining of the inside of her uterus. The surgery went smoothly and there were no complications.

Shanitra was very pleased with the almost invisible scar and even happier to learn that she could give birth without needing a Cesarean. Since my incision in her uterus was done in such a way as to avoid going into the cavity, a vaginal birth was safe. She waited the three months I advised in order to heal and then began to try again for a baby. Three months after that, she came to see me: she was still not pregnant and was worried because they'd conceived almost immediately in their prior pregnancies. She recalled the information I'd given her during that meeting months ago—that 10 percent of women develop scarring after surgery and that it can prevent conception. Was she part of this 10 percent, she wondered, and should she be worried?

I told her that only 50 percent of patients who are attempting pregnancy with no history of surgery, miscarriage, or any other malady will conceive in six months of trying. So, even when there are no problems, that small window of opportunity each month when a woman can conceive is just that—small. The likelihood was that everything was within the normal time frame and nothing was necessarily wrong, since her examination and sonogram were totally normal at this visit. I advised her to be optimistic and continue trying for pregnancy, but to come back if she was not pregnant in the next three months. At that point, I would do further testing just to be sure there were no surprises. I could see this gave Shanitra a little relief and, armed with the statistics that were on her side, she left my office cautiously hopeful.

One month later she missed her period and the home pregnancy test was positive. Initially, Shanitra was thrilled, but then nervousness set in: What if something went wrong again? What if her body began to produce another fibroid tumor? After all, the one before was large and she didn't even know it was there. Could another one grow without her knowing? I answered her questions: pregnancy can cause fibroids to grow, and I would watch for it, but it most likely would not get big enough to cause a problem. Meanwhile, there was none that I could find, either by examination or sonogram. All of her initial tests were normal. I followed her closely through her pregnancy and, except for nausea and vomiting making her feel pretty awful for the first three months, she sailed right through her pregnancy. No new fibroids appeared on her monthly sonograms, and her baby grew normally. After a long labor and lots of pushing, she delivered Tasha, a gorgeous 7 lb 2 oz girl, without a problem and to the great delight of the new parents and grandmother. Since then, Shanitra went on to have another healthy pregnancy. I delivered her second daughter, Brenda, three years later, and so far there are still no new fibroids. The only thing Shanitra was growing in her uterus was cute little girls.

## WHAT ARE FIBROIDS?

Fibroid tumors are the most common tumors of the uterus. No one knows how many women actually have them—Shanitra went through three miscarriages before hers was discovered—and they usually cause only minor symptoms so they often go unrecognized. Sometimes they can cause heavy menstrual flow and pain (like Shanitra's after she stopped taking her oral contraceptives), depending on their location in the uterus and their size.

In some women, fibroids can cause miscarriage. Although they are considered a tumor, they are not cancerous and become cancerous only very rarely: less than 1 in 1,000 will become malignant. So, unless there is unusually rapid growth, these tumors will not require immediate attention. They can be left in place to be removed only when they cause symptoms.

Each fibroid arises from a single cell in the muscular wall of the uterus. These tumors are really muscle cell tumors and are not fibroid under a microscope, but look fibrous when seen by the unaided eye. They are sensitive to estrogen and progesterone, the normal female hormones. They will grow in response to these hormones during the normal menstrual cycle, when taking oral contraceptive pills, and during pregnancy.

In pregnancy these hormones reach through-the-roof levels, so fibroids can grow to huge proportions. They may cause pain, preterm labor, and—as in Shanitra's case—miscarriage. What makes them tricky is that when the pregnancy is over, they will shrink, becoming much smaller. Because of this, they may not be recognized as the cause of the problem when the doctor is seeking a diagnosis between miscarriages.

## WHAT CAN BE DONE

Ultrasound and pelvic examinations are helpful in formulating the diagnosis. A saline infusion sonohysterogram or hysterosalpingogram (see Chapter 9) can help in diagnosis. Hysteroscopy (see Chapter 5) will be helpful, as well, usually combined with **laparoscopic surgery**. The laparoscopic approach, a minimally invasive **endoscopic** procedure, can often be used for treatment in addition to diagnosis. If the fibroids are not too large and not too close to the major blood vessels of the uterus, the tumor or tumors can be removed by laparoscopic surgery using two or three small incisions in the abdominal wall. Usually there is a one-centimeter incision through the navel, with lasers or other laparoscopic instruments inserted through the incisions and viewed on a TV monitor attached to a telescope-like instrument. When the fibroids are within the cavity of the uterus they can be removed vaginally through the hysteroscope using a special instrument called a resectoscope, also attached to a TV camera, which has an electrical loop to remove things with minimal blood loss.

## laparoscopic surgery

Considered a minimally invasive procedure, laparoscopic surgery is performed by making several small incisions in the abdomen, usually one-half to one centimeter in length. An incision is made through the navel (although the incision may also be made just below the navel, I like to make it through the navel so the scar can't be seen). A thin, long tube called a laparoscope is inserted through the incision into the patient. A camera is attached to the outside of the laparoscope, enabling the surgeon to see inside the patient by viewing an image on a TV screen transmitted by the camera. Tiny instruments are then inserted through secondary incisions to perform the surgery.

## endoscopy

Using a telescopic instrument to visualize structures within the body.

There are other minimally invasive procedures that have been used with success for treatment of fibroids also, including:

- *Uterine artery embolization.* A procedure in which a radiologist uses fluoroscopic guidance with real-time X-rays on a monitor to pass a thin tube into a uterine artery through the main artery in the leg. The doctor then injects a substance that will close off the uterine artery and destroy the blood supply to the uterus in the area of the injection. This will cause the fibroids to die and the uterus to shrink in size.

- *Radio-frequency ablation.* A fine needle is inserted under ultrasound or fluoroscopic guidance, or occasionally through laparoscopy, into the fibroid, and a high-frequency current is used to destroy the tumor. There is very little information available about using uterine artery embolization and radio-frequency ablation as a treatment for recurrent miscarriage.

Both of these procedures are new and not widely used as of yet for treatment of recurrent miscarriage. While they may well be valuable in the future when there is more information available, right now they are used for treating fibroids that are causing excess bleeding in women who are good candidates for minimally invasive surgery, or not interested in pregnancy, or not good risks for major surgery.

Presently, the gold standard for large fibroids is myomectomy with complete removal of the offending fibroid tumors, as I performed on Shanitra. After removal of the fibroids, the uterus has to heal well enough to support a term pregnancy. I usually recommend a minimum of three months' healing time, during which pregnancy is not attempted and condoms are used as a couple's form of contraception. Remember: the hormones in birth control pills may contribute to the growth of fibroids. By that point, the uterus has healed and it is safe for a couple to begin trying again.

In order for a vaginal birth to be safe, the surgery used to remove the fibroid tumor(s) should not enter the lining of the inside of the womb. If this cavity is cut into when the surgery is performed to remove the fibroids, then the full thickness of the wall of the uterus has been cut through. It is believed that this creates a weak spot in healing that could rupture under the stress of labor. In those cases most surgeons recommend a Cesarean birth rather than an attempted vaginal delivery. Either way, once the fibroids are gone a normal, full-term pregnancy and a healthy baby are the usual result. An accurate diagnosis and skillfully performed surgery can make all the difference for a woman with uterine fibroids.

# thirteen

## MULTIPLE PREGNANCY: LESS IS MORE

~~~~~~~~~~~~~~~~~~~~~~~~~~~~~~~~~~~~~~~~~~~~~~~

## LUCILLE

IT WAS AN URGENT CALL FROM ONE OF OUR OB/GYN nurses, and I took it immediately. Although none of my hospitalized high-risk patients had a problem, you never can tell about the unexpected. Luckily, it was not that kind of a call. The nurse just wanted me to see her brother's wife for a fertility problem, and, of course, I agreed.

Her sister-in-law, Lucille, was 27 years old and a petite five feet two inches tall, with straight black hair and almost black eyes. Her husband, Nelson, entered my office first, sitting in the chair closest to the door. "Scoot in, honey," I remember her jokingly saying to Nelson as she squeezed her slightly chubby frame past him for the other seat. Nelson stood his muscular five-foot-ten-inch frame up immediately, apologizing profusely and allowing his wife to pass. Despite his tough-looking demeanor, complete with a gold loop earring in each ear and a shaved head, when it came to Lucille, Nelson was a teddy bear. He was an assistant building superintendent on the Upper East Side of Manhattan, he told me, eyeing me dubiously as the smile for his wife left his face. I could not help thinking of the Mr. Clean commercial after I had met him.

Lucille told me that she worked in the administration department of a Catholic school in the same neighborhood in which her husband worked. It was a great arrangement that allowed them to travel to and from work together. And, because she was an employee, their kids could attend Lucille's school at a discounted tuition, even though they weren't parishioners. It was an ideal situation that was missing one obvious, key component: the kids. After years of trying she couldn't seem to get pregnant, Lucille told me sadly.

After doing the history and physical exam, I had a good idea of Lucille's problem. Her menstrual periods were two, sometimes three, months apart and she had increased hair on her upper lip, around her nipples, and on her tummy. On pelvic examination, her ovaries were enlarged and felt cystic (fluid filled). An ultrasound examination showed **polycystic ovaries,** and her blood tests confirmed the diagnosis. Nelson's sperm count showed that he was fertile, so we knew what the problem was, but nothing is as easy as it looks.

---

### polycystic ovary syndrome (pco)

A condition in which the ovaries are enlarged and filled with fluid cysts and do not ovulate. There is a high degree of male hormone present and the patient is often overweight and infertile.

---

## OVERCOMING THE PROBLEM

Treatment with the usual clomiphene, a drug used to induce ovulation, did not make Lucille ovulate, even in high doses; neither did metformin, another drug used for the same purpose. After six months of treatment, Lucille was getting upset and impatient. Nelson demanded to know why the treatment did not work. Not only that, but they wanted to know why I was not doing more. I know how intensely upsetting infertility is for any patient who experiences it, and that it's not uncommon for them to turn to (and sometimes feel angry at) their doctor when their frustration boils over. I patiently explained to the young couple that changing her ovulation drugs could put Lucille at increased risk of **ovarian hyperstimulation syndrome (OHSS), ovarian torsion,** and multiple pregnancy, which is more common for patients who have the PCO syndrome. The risks are known to increase with higher doses of drugs, especially with injections of gonadotropin drugs, which stimulate the ovary vigorously. I combined the treatment using metformin continuously and a maximum dose of clomiphene, followed by an injection of chorionic gonadotropin. Still no luck.

---

## ovarian hyperstimulation syndrome (ohss)

OHSS occurs when drugs used to induce ovulation cause rapid enlargement of the ovarian cysts and fluid accumulates in them, as well as inside the abdominal cavity. This causes a drop in the patient's circulating blood volume and may lead to low blood pressure and shock.

---

## ovarian torsion

The ovary and usually the oviduct twist, and their blood supply gets blocked, often causing severe abdominal pain and death of the ovary and oviduct.

---

When Lucille and Nelson heard "multiple pregnancies," they looked at each other, their eyes growing wide, and said simultaneously, "That would be great!" They'd been trying for so long that having twins, or even triplets, sounded wonderful. Why, they asked, could this be considered a bad thing?

I explained: About one out of three patients treated with gonadotropins have twins, about one in ten have triplets, and one in a hundred have more than three babies. And while this might seem, to some parents, like a winning situation, it is not without serious

considerations. Multiple pregnancies come with several complications, as does caring for twins and for triplets. Prematurity and fetal loss are a major problem. Treatment for such pregnancies can
even be dangerous to both the mother's and babies' health. Lucille
and Nelson looked at each other again and began talking it over.
Nelson was worried about Lucille's safety; Lucille did not care. It
did not seem so risky to her. At last Lucille said, "I think we should
go for it." Nelson grabbed his wife's hand and nodded his head in
agreement. Lucille looked at me and said, "I want to do whatever it
takes." What else could I say but okay?

I was still very cautious. I gave Lucille only a moderate dose of
clomiphene followed by five consecutive days of a low dose (75
units) of gonadotropin, watching her closely. I followed her estradiol hormone levels to monitor the development of the **ovarian
follicles** that produce it, and sonograms to see the size and the
number of ovarian follicles. There were four ripe follicles on cycle
day 14. At that point I gave her a dose of 5,000 units of human
chorionic gonadotropin to trigger ovulation on cycle day 15 or 16. I
told Lucille to be sure that Nelson stayed home that night; in fact,
maybe for the next two or three nights. Now was the time for the
couple to try again for a pregnancy.

---

### ovarian follicle
A roundish cavity that contains fluid and a maturing egg, or
ovum, and is surrounded by a layer of cells.

---

Three weeks later, Lucille had a positive home pregnancy
test. One week after that I had three pregnancy sacs on the sonogram. Lucille was beside herself with astonishment and excitement.
"Triplets?! You're not serious!?" she exclaimed in the examining
room. I explained that it was too soon to be sure. We'll see in two

weeks, I said. Two weeks later, though, during our next sonogram there were only two embryos on the screen; one had disappeared. I could see by Lucille's expression that she was stricken by this news. When she'd entered my office that day, she'd had a tentative smile on her face and said, "Let's see how we're doing today." As is sometimes the case with many expecting moms after a sonogram, Lucille felt like she was already bonding with the embryos inside her. She knew that she might lose an embryo early in the pregnancy, as I had warned. I wanted her to remain unbonded until the situation was clear. Still, the lost embryo pained her.

"Is it my fault?" she said to me. "Somehow I feel that it is. Did I do anything to make this happen?" I explained: "Definitely NO," that it was not unusual, and that this was referred to as **vanishing twin syndrome,** a spontaneous loss of one embryo in a multiple pregnancy that usually occurs in the first three months. It disappears completely and is absorbed, because it is the least healthy of the embryos.

---

### vanishing twin syndrome
The spontaneous loss of one embryo in a multiple pregnancy in the first three months. It usually disappears completely and is absorbed.

---

What was unusual in this case, though, was that the sonogram showed that the remaining twins were one-egg identical twins (**monozygotic**). Usually, in two out of three cases, the twins are from two different eggs, which are called fraternal (dizygotic) twins. Not only did the best egg win, it split and reproduced itself after fertilization in Lucille's pregnancy. Miscarriage is more common with twins, but even more so with one-egg twins, because of more abnormal fetuses and **placentas,** and greater demands for oxygen and nutrients in multiple pregnancies. So even more intensive monitoring was needed for Lucille's pregnancy.

---

## monozygotic (identical) twins

Twins that come from a single fertilized egg and are almost always mirror images of each other. Their placentas are fused, but they can vary in the amount of blood supply per twin, as well as in weight or abnormalities.

---

She was followed closely, and she was fine until 24 weeks of pregnancy when she felt her uterus contracting and those contractions persisted for one or two hours every afternoon. An examination and a sonogram showed that her cervix was thinning out earlier than it should. It also showed that the twins were boys. Baby A was about 25 percent bigger than baby B on the sonogram, also. Since they were identical twins from one egg, they had to be of the same sex, but usually one-egg twins are close to the same size. But in Lucille's pregnancy, baby B was lagging behind due to limited placental function. If that problem continued and became severe, baby B could outgrow his already reduced placental blood supply and die. If one identical twin is lost, the surviving twin will die soon afterward in 25 percent of all cases; up to 50 percent of the remaining survivors will have brain damage.

At this point, it was crucial to keep a close eye on the twins with ultrasound every week, and keep Lucille at bed rest and off work. I explained to the couple that an early delivery was likely. I had to prevent preterm birth too early, but time it before we lost one of the babies. The tests of fetal well-being—biophysical profiles and umbilical artery **Doppler studies**—were done twice a week. Every two weeks cervical length and fetal weight were estimated by ultrasound.

doppler study

An ultrasound technique to measure blood flow used for the umbilical artery or the middle cerebral artery to determine the blood flow between the fetus and placenta or the blood flow in the baby's brain.

Baby B kept losing ground, though. By 33 weeks of pregnancy, he was only 60 percent of his brother. His biophysical profile score fell to six out of ten, into the risky zone for fetal loss with a decrease in amniotic fluid and fewer fetal movements. Also, the Doppler showed absent end diastolic blood flow, which is a sign of poor blood flow between the baby and the placenta reducing the baby's oxygen and nutrition. There was more danger to the baby from waiting than from prematurity. It was time for delivery.

At 34 weeks and 1 day, I performed a Cesarean delivery of the twins, baby B first, Leon, at 3 lb 2 oz. Louis, the second baby, weighed in at 5 lb 6 oz. Despite his smaller size, Leon was the tough guy, older by two minutes; small but scrappy. Louis, bigger, but second born, had some mild breathing problems due to what is called respiratory distress syndrome. This happens when a baby's lungs aren't mature enough at birth. In the case of Lucille's twins, Leon's stressful experience of declining placental function had actually sped up his lungs' development, compensating him for the lost weight by maturing him faster than his bigger, but younger by two minutes, brother. Louis's lungs rapidly responded to treatment by the neonatal staff, and by his third day of life he needed no help in breathing. Both boys soon went home to their mom and dad, and were thriving when I next saw them at six weeks old. I kept in touch and followed their progress over the last seven years. Believe it or not, they were featured in several magazine advertisements.

Leon is still smaller and thinner than Louis, but he remains the dominant big brother over his "identical" twin.

## WHAT CAUSES MULTIPLE PREGNANCY LOSS?

Every culture has myths about twins, varying from the Yoruba tribe in West Africa, who believe that twins are one person split in two by Shango, the thunder god; to Italians, some of whom still tell the tale that Romulus and Remus were raised by a wolf to found the ancient city of Rome. But myths aside, there are risks attached to multiple pregnancy of which expecting parents aren't always aware. And with the new fertility drugs and the technological advances in reproductive medicine, we are seeing an explosive increase in multiple births: the incidence of twins has more than doubled in the last 20 years and triplets have increased sixfold.

For the mother, there is a greater frequency of maternal problems, such as high blood pressure, diabetes, and bleeding from the placenta. There are also other problems:

- A higher pregnancy loss rate as miscarriage occurs about twice as often in twins than it does for single-fetus pregnancies. About 30 percent of twin pregnancies will miscarry, and this is true in all three trimesters of pregnancy. This is in addition to the vanishing twin syndrome, as in Lucille's case.
- A higher rate of preterm labor and premature birth is a major problem, as well as a higher frequency of abnormal fetuses, **discordant twins** and the ensuing problems they experience, and the rare but serious problem of twin-to-twin transfusion syndrome.

---

### discordant twins

Twins that differ by at least 20 percent in weight. This can be accompanied by other differences such as in gender, abnormalities, and placentas.

---

When dealing with multiples, especially triplets or more, the greatest risk to the babies is preterm birth that results in loss of the newborn. With these high-order multiple pregnancies, it is very likely that an extremely immature newborn will be unable to survive outside the womb because of difficulties with respiratory distress syndrome and failure of the immature body to function properly. Dealing with this kind of multiple pregnancy is an extremely delicate matter, and one that will require close monitoring by and cooperation with your physician. Some of the other problems that may be encountered with multiple pregnancy that can lead to pregnancy loss are not common, but occur often enough that you need to know about them when thinking about miscarriage and multiple pregnancies.

### Vanishing Twin Syndrome

It's not a stretch to say that competition for survival among human beings begins in the womb, and vanishing twin syndrome is a prime example. The vanishing twin syndrome is a problem that occurs more often than we actually know because it can be recognized only by early and frequent sonograms. It is estimated to occur in 36 percent of twins, 53 percent of triplets, and 65 percent of quadruplets when the diagnosis is made by sonogram. Why does it happen? The vanished twin is thought to be an abnormal embryo, unable to survive in the early competitive environment of multiple pregnancy.

Similarly, the early miscarriages with twins or more are thought to be from abnormal embryos, which are usually the weakest. When there is just so much blood flow and just so much room for a placenta, the weakest embryos cannot survive. But, later on, the placenta can still play a pivotal role in the survival of twins. For fraternal twins, differences in placental size and function can cause the loss of one of the twins. If the twins are identical, differences in blood flow to their shared placenta may cause pregnancy loss of both identical twins as in twin-to-twin transfusion syndrome. With triplets or more, placental competition for blood flow may result in pregnancy loss or neonatal death for the fetus with the least placental support. With many twins, and with triplets or higher, there is also an increased incidence of preterm birth, sometimes two months early.

### Twin-to-Twin Transfusion Syndrome

Although it's seen in only about 10 to 20 percent of one-egg twins, twin-to-twin transfusion syndrome is another potential complication of multiple pregnancy. At birth for most twins, the oxygen level and chemistry in the blood favors the firstborn, no matter how it is delivered, and the firstborn is usually more vigorous at birth. But, with twin-to-twin transfusion syndrome, one fetus is the donor, sharing its placental blood flow with its twin, who greedily sucks up oxygen and nutrition from its donor twin's blood. The result may be a disaster for both, with the death of one twin in 60 percent of instances, and loss of both twins in 20 percent of all cases of twin-to-twin transfusion syndrome. If one survives, about half of those surviving twins will have neurological abnormalities such as cerebral palsy. When twin-to-twin transfusion syndrome occurs, the donor baby is at least 20 to 25 percent smaller. That baby has a decreased amount of amniotic fluid (called oligohydramnios), while the recipient has an excessive amount of amniotic fluid (called polyhydramnios). The donor can die from lack of oxygen and low blood volume, going into shock. The recipient can die from heart failure from an overloaded circulation. If one dies, the theory is that the survivor bleeds into the dead fetus through their shared placental blood circulations. Shock results and then death or brain damage of the survivor.

If the diagnosis is made early then treatment is possible, and there are several courses your doctor can take:

- *Serial amniocentesis.* This removes excessive amniotic fluid (polyhydramnios) and reduces it from the sac of the recipient in order to try to save both twins.
- *Fetoscopic laser surgery.* This coagulates the communicating blood vessels connecting the twins' blood flow in the placenta that is shared by the two fetuses. This separates their blood circulations from each other in an attempt to save both twins.
- *Umbilical cord coagulation.* If an abnormality is present in one twin, or that twin is already dying and cannot be saved, coagulating, or stopping the blood flow, in the umbilical cord of the abnormal twin will stop the transfusion process and prevent blood loss into a dead fetus from the healthy one, and thus save the latter.

## Twin-Reversed Arterial Perfusion Syndrome

Another variation of this problem of connecting blood vessels between twins is twin-reversed arterial perfusion syndrome (TRAP), which happens rarely—only 1 percent of all multiple pregnancies. When this does occur, one twin is abnormal with malformations, such as an absent chest or head, and no functional heart. The other twin pumps blood for the abnormal one and for itself. The excessive work on the heart of the normal twin leads to death of both in 55 percent of cases and possible brain damage if the normal twin survives. Umbilical cord coagulation or early delivery can save the normal twin.

## Monoamniotic Twins

Monoamniotic twins are one-egg twins (identical) where there is one big placenta and one sac instead of a sac for each fetus. The split of the fertilized egg occurs 8 to 13 days after fertilization, relatively late in embryonic life. This creates a problem in which the two umbilical cords can become tangled, causing fetal death of one or both twins in 10 to 54 percent of cases. However, monoamniotic twins occur in less than 1 percent of one-egg twins—a very rare occurrence, indeed. This type of pregnancy loss requires close observation in the hospital after 26 weeks, and delivery around 32 to 34 weeks instead of the full 40 weeks of pregnancy if the babies are to be saved.

## Pregnancy Reduction

This is performed in late first trimester and early second trimester under ultrasound guidance by injecting a drug that stops the fetal heart into one or more fetuses. This is sometimes offered with triplets or higher. It carries about a 5 to 8 percent risk of losing the whole pregnancy from the procedure. The issues of **multifetal pregnancy reduction** and **selective termination** are very complex and should be discussed with your doctor where they might be a consideration.

---

### multifetal pregnancy reduction

Partial abortion of one or more fetuses, preserving the rest in order to continue the pregnancy and decrease the risk of preterm births.

---

---

### selective termination

Selective termination is a form of multifetal pregnancy reduction when there is one abnormal fetus, which can be aborted, leaving the normal fetus to continue the pregnancy.

---

## WHAT CAN BE DONE?

Much has changed in modern science to the benefit of multiple births, although it is still a road with miscarriage risk and problems. Sonography early in the first trimester of pregnancy is now almost universal and greatly improves our ability for early diagnosis—the biggest key to treatment and care for multiple pregnancy. When two sacs are seen on a sonogram, it is still only a 57 percent chance that the twins will actually be born because of the vanishing twin syndrome. However, if there is a good, strong heartbeat in both sacs at 8 weeks (120 to 180 beats per minute), those odds go up to 87 percent. With three sacs, it is only a 20 percent survival rate for triplets, but that statistic rises to 68 percent if all have normal heartbeats in the 120 to 180 beats per minute range at 8 weeks.

Another advantage that sonography allows is that we can almost always tell if there are two-egg twins using sonograms, and this is very important in the management of multiple pregnancy. When dealing with triplets and higher, 33 weeks at preterm birth is expected for 90 percent, but twins will usually go to 37 weeks or more with careful management. A big part of properly handling a multiple pregnancy is knowing exactly what we're dealing with—a key piece of knowledge that sonography affords.

Multiples can be followed by serial sonograms for growth and discordancy. Sonograms also allow us to measure cervical length for evidence of an increased risk of preterm birth. With a more than 25 percent rate of discordancy for multiples, pregnancy loss of one or both twins is increased by six and a half times. This is why it is vital to measure and evaluate fetal growth every two to three weeks. Sonograms also allow us to look for complications like twin-to-twin transfusion syndrome. When such problems arise, carefully timed delivery, as in Lucille's case, with specific treatment for other kinds of complications, can be performed.

Modern medicine also allows us to screen for maternal complications earlier in pregnancy than ever before. Some of the things we keep an eye on because they are more frequent in multiples are high blood pressure, diabetes, and abnormal location of the placenta causing bleeding. Care of the patient with twin-to-twin transfusion syndrome, TRAP, and monoamniotic twins, as well as triplets and higher, must be individualized with comprehensive counseling about the risks and alternatives and the likelihood of preterm delivery. Such patients need specialized care with maternal-fetal medicine physicians, neonatologists, and a team approach to their complex situation.

We can also use the same tests to diagnose genetic problems that we use for singletons. However, prenatal genetic diagnosis for multiples is a bit more complicated because blood test results are normally higher than what is seen in a singleton pregnancy and must be interpreted differently. The good news: chromosome defects in multiple pregnancy are not increased compared with chromosome defects in singletons. Still, the tests for genetic diagnosis become more complicated—amniocenteses for two-egg twins will require sampling *each* sac, and **chorionic villus sampling (CVS)**, will require sampling more than one fetus.

---

## chorionic villus sampling (cvs)

A genetic test performed at 10 to 12 weeks of pregnancy where a minuscule piece of the placenta is biopsied in order to detect abnormalities with a fetus early.

Another important factor in this equation is you—being a responsible patient is important. One of the things you must do is keep a close watch over your nutritional needs. For instance, your folic acid is increased to 1 mg and your iron intake from 60 mg to 320 mg per day. You also need to consume at least a 2,200-calorie diet, since more nutrition and vitamins are necessary with multiple pregnancy. More babies means more nutrition is required and expect more weight gain. Also, by 20 to 28 weeks, many doctors recommend decreased activity for multiple pregnancy patients to reduce the chance of preterm birth. If your physician tells you to get off your feet, do it! I understand that with two-family incomes, household responsibilities, and just the general demands of adult life, this is not as easy (or fun) as it sounds. But if your doctor prescribes bed rest, take that order as seriously as you would medication. It can make a difference of several weeks of fetal development when preterm birth seems likely.

Multiple pregnancy is a high-risk situation, and special care is needed for such women. In spite of all these problems the outlook has never been better for multiple-pregnancy patients. Just look around you at the double and triple baby strollers every time you take a walk in the park. There is much more success these days for moms pregnant with multiples because the technology is available, and because patients are much better informed. Having a strong, trusting, cooperative relationship with your doctor is vital, too. And remember: you might think that the work of being a parent of multiple babies begins after they're born—but it really starts in the womb.

# section three

~~~~~~~~~~~~~~~~~~~~~~~~~~~~~~~~~~~~~~~~~~~~~~~~

MALFUNCTIONS: SYSTEMS FAILURE

# fourteen

## SEVERE MATERNAL ILLNESS: BLINDSIDED

~~~~~~~~~~~~~~~~~~~~~~~~~~~~~~~~~~~~~~~~~~~~~~

## MARIA THERESA

A TALL, ELEGANT, AND BEAUTIFUL WOMAN ENTERED MY office and offered me her hand. Her name was Maria Theresa and she was five feet ten inches tall with reddish-brown hair and gray-green eyes. Even when she took a seat it was graceful—she moved precisely like the dancer she was. She and her husband, Juan, who accompanied her that day, were a professional flamenco dance team performing mostly on cruise ships and in an occasional nightclub in between cruises. Juan was the embodiment of the male flamenco dancer concept: six feet tall, black hair, dark-brown eyes, and chiseled, aquiline features. They looked more like they belonged at a café in Andalusia than sitting across from me in my office at NYU Medical Center. I shook Juan's hand and asked them to tell me what their problem was. It was a terrible story, the kind that leaves you speechless and awed.

Maria had been pregnant on one of the cruises and had not been feeling at all well. By the fourth month, she was very nauseated, had a constant headache, and her middle was starting to bulge. When the ship arrived in the port of Sydney, Australia, she saw a doctor. He told her that she had very high blood pressure and needed to be in the hospital. He said that she could lose the baby or have a stroke. She was only 18 weeks pregnant.

The ship was going to sail out of Sydney at six P.M. and she and Juan had to decide whether to stay and be hospitalized in Australia

or continue on the ship and live up to their contract. The cruise
would be over in five days and then they could fly home to
Barcelona and get medical care from the doctors they knew in
Spain. They stayed aboard ship and took the first flight home to
Barcelona. She somehow tolerated her symptoms, but she was
grateful that there was only one more performance for them. The
day they arrived back, they called the doctor in Barcelona and were
told he could see them in one week. Eager to take the first opening
he had, Maria and Juan agreed to the date, not believing that anything bad could happen to them, she said.

Maria told me that she tried to console herself during that
time. She convinced herself that what she was experiencing was
normal. Lots of women continued to be nauseated into their second trimester. Hers, however, began during that period—still, she
and Juan wanted to remain calm, and they did. Maria and Juan
canceled their dance practices for the next week, figuring it couldn't
hurt to take it a little easy, and she was uncharacteristically tired
anyway.

She saw the doctor at 20 weeks of pregnancy. Juan went with
her; he was worried. She was nervous, she told me, but hoped the
visit would just be the doctor advising more rest. After she arrived,
the physician performed an ultrasound. At this point in our conversation, Maria stopped talking and looked down at the floor,
creasing her forehead at the horrific memory she was trying to describe. Tears swelled from her eyes, and Juan reached over and
gently took her hand. She took a deep breath and shook her head,
signaling to him that she couldn't continue telling the story. Juan
looked away from his wife to me, and muttered what she couldn't
say: "The ultrasound showed that our baby was dead."

Maria was taken right to the hospital with very high blood
pressure, given intravenous medication, and the rest was a blur in
her mind after that. The baby, a little girl, was born dead, and
Maria was sent home two days later with blood pressure medication. She was told never to try pregnancy again or she would die.

She was done grieving and wanted a baby, she said. That was one year before this visit.

## OVERCOMING THE PROBLEM

Despite the harrowing experience of her first pregnancy, and the fact that her doctor in Barcelona told her that she was likely to lose her own life if she tried, Maria did indeed desperately want to try again. During my career, I have seen women perform some amazing feats of strength in order to have children, and Maria was certainly one of them. She was 34 and Juan was only 28, which she admitted was another factor in her urgency. "I have to give him a child," she told me during our visit, "it wouldn't be fair..." She trailed off, seeming to not know exactly which part of "not fair" to peg this on. And that was when she dropped it on me: "I am two months pregnant," she told me in a matter-of-fact tone, and shrugged her shoulders. Juan squirmed in his chair and said nothing; his wife had made up her mind and he seemed to know there wasn't much he could do to talk her out of it.

I continued taking her medical history, which was significant in that her mother and sister both had high blood pressure. At this visit, her blood pressure was 140/90, too high to be normal, but not as bad as I had expected. Her examination, however, revealed two large structures in her abdomen where her kidneys should be—but they weren't odd, foreign objects, they *were* her kidneys. Her uterus was the right size for an eight-week pregnancy, but her kidneys were huge. An ultrasound exam confirmed an eight-week fetus with a good heartbeat. It also showed that both her kidneys were enlarged and filled with multiple fluid-filled sacs. She had polycystic kidney disease, clearly the source of her high blood pressure and the reason for the miscarriage of her first pregnancy.

Now that I had the diagnosis, further testing had to be done to determine how severe her kidney disease actually was. The news was not good at all: the full range of tests showed severe polycystic kidney disease at the most advanced stage. My review of the medical literature showed that there had never been a case of fetal survival when it was this bad. Not only that, but nine out of the ten women who tried pregnancy with this severe kidney disease had died along with the fetus. At our meeting two weeks later, I explained this very serious news to Maria and Juan. After her ultrasound revealed a ten-week living fetus with a strong heartbeat on the screen, there was no thought of anything else. She didn't even hesitate: she was going to have this baby, and she would risk her life for it, she told me. I went over all the risks to her and her baby and confirmed that her mind was made up. Then I said, "If you have the courage to do this, I have to be brave enough to go through it with you."

I started her on medicine to control her blood pressure immediately, as well as a high-calorie and low-protein diet, because her kidneys could not handle the protein but she needed calories for fetal growth. We made it to six months without hospitalization. We were two-thirds of the way there when Maria's condition began to seriously affect her health. First, I had to put her in the hospital to control her blood pressure. From that point forward, things were very tense, with Maria in the hospital on bed rest for the remainder of the pregnancy. She also had to be on a salt- and protein-restricted diet because her kidneys were working at only 10 percent of normal. Too much salt would raise her blood pressure and too much protein could not be removed by her kidneys, causing poisoning of the fetus. In addition, I had to very closely monitor her response to the blood pressure medication, which needed to be increased again and again.

Even with all this careful monitoring and planning, sonograms showed that the baby's growth was slowing. A biophysical profile showed the fetus to be well at 32 weeks. However, when we got to 7 weeks before her due date, her blood pressure began climbing again uncontrollably and the baby stopped growing. There was no choice; I had to deliver Maria. She understood, and her will for a baby was stronger than ever. Her life and her baby were now in real danger and we both knew it.

I gave her two doses of dexamethasone 12 hours apart, a drug that helps to trigger the baby's lungs to develop and prevent it from having breathing problems because it was much too early to be born. The next two days of waiting for the fetal lungs' development to speed up from the medication were nerve-racking for all of us. Could mother and baby get through them without a disaster and hang in there long enough for me to time delivery just right?

At 33 weeks and 5 days of pregnancy, with the mother on huge doses of medication to control her blood pressure, I delivered a baby boy via Cesarean with epidural anesthesia: tiny, but healthy. He weighed only four pounds, but he breathed and cried vigorously. He was determined to live, maybe with the same kind of strength as his mom. When she heard him, Maria Theresa cried, too—the first time I saw her cry since that first day in my office; but this time, they were beautiful tears of joy, the best kind. And when Juan realized that Maria was fine, and so was his son, he began crying, too—huge sobs of relief and happiness after the incredibly tense and frightening six months they both endured.

Maria Theresa recovered very slowly, but she did finally get back to her pre-pregnancy state by three months after her Cesarean. However, her kidneys progressively failed. Three years after delivering little Sebastian, she was still unable to work. Her career was over, but she had Sebastian to care for. Somehow she looked after him in between maintaining their home and dialysis three times a week. Two years after she began dialysis, she finally got a kidney transplant in the United States. Her son was five years old, a normal, healthy, little boy, and the joy of her and Juan's life. She never gave up and she never regretted her choice.

## WHAT CAUSES SEVERE MATERNAL ILLNESS?

When a woman has a serious medical problem, miscarriage is a frequent occurrence if she overcomes the not uncommon infertility and becomes pregnant. Mother Nature seems most willing to give up the fetus rather than the life of the mother. If there is a very severe disease, both may be lost. It is no small risk and something you should not enter into without a thorough discussion with your partner and your doctor. That is, of course, why many doctors advise against pregnancy for women with severe illness, just as Maria Theresa's doctor in Barcelona did. She chose to risk her life to have her child. She had severe kidney disease to a potentially fatal degree. My practice is always to explain, to offer choices based on risks and possible outcomes, and to let my patients make their own informed decisions. Even if I had wanted to, by the time she entered my office, I didn't have the option to advise her against pregnancy—she was already pregnant. I had to do everything I could to keep her and her baby healthy and alive through pregnancy and delivery.

Maria Theresa had a great result. When the result is not good the support system is really necessary. The emotional burden of a dangerous pregnancy needs sharing. Shared with spouse, family, friends, physician, and clergy, the burden is spread and more tolerable. Except for the doctor, who carries the awesome responsibility for two lives: mother and child in one failing body.

Fortunately, modern medical care was able to carry Maria Theresa through her pregnancy and bring her a healthy child. This is, of course, something you have on your side (as with all of the conditions discussed in this book): today's medicine has made childbearing possible for many women who thought that they could never have a baby. Women with severe kidney or liver disease are just one example, but there are many other conditions, such as:

heart disease
lung disease

auto-immune disease
intestinal disease
diabetes
high blood pressure
cancers
patients at high risk for stroke
spinal cord injury with paralysis
sickle cell and other anemias

Each one carries risk to the mother's life and well-being, varying with severity of the illness. Each carries some increased risk for miscarriage, especially with acute flare-ups of the disease. These women must have careful treatment before, during, and after pregnancy. If you know you have any of these conditions, it is of the utmost importance that you consult with your doctor before attempting pregnancy so you are fully aware of the risks to your health, to the health of your potential baby, and to your family.

## WHAT CAN BE DONE

First and foremost, in order to treat an illness it must be diagnosed. A pre-conceptional visit to your doctor and appropriate laboratory tests and counseling based on your age, medical history, and physical examination will go a long way toward knowing that you have a problem. After it is correctly diagnosed, your physician can treat your condition. Once it is controlled and stable with appropriate medication and therapy, pregnancy can usually be undertaken—however, I urge you to be clear on the risks involved. There is certainly much to be said for blind faith—it gets people through all kinds of difficult trials in life—but denial is another matter. Pretending your condition doesn't exist is a dangerous path for any mother and baby. The patient must be counseled about the risks of pregnancy to her own life and the life of her child, which may well include a high risk of death or disability to both of them.

These risks vary depending on the severity of the illness and how pregnancy affects the disease, as well as how the disease affects the pregnancy. Usually, a maternal/fetal medicine specialist and the patient's medical doctor must collaborate in the care of the pregnant woman and her fetus. In some cases, a specialist in care of the newborn must be consulted when there is a significant risk of a preterm birth or potential disability for the baby. Once pregnancy occurs, *very close monitoring* of the mother-to-be and her fetus is required.

Specific tests for the mother's condition must be performed related directly to the nature of her illness, as well as tests of fetal well-being. At appropriate intervals, these tests have to be repeated more and more frequently as term approaches. These fetal tests include:

- Fetal heart rate monitoring with what is called a **nonstress test**
- Ultrasounds done periodically to assess fetal growth
- The biophysical profile to evaluate fetal condition
- **Doppler studies** of the umbilical artery and middle cerebral artery of the fetus

---

### nonstress test
A fetal heart rate test to evaluate fetal well-being by observing increases in the fetal heart rate associated with fetal movements.

---

Of course, there can be many other tests depending on specific fetal risks. The goal is delivery at or close to full term, although sometimes that is just not attainable, as with Maria Theresa. Her son, Sebastian, stopped growing in her womb at eight months. A Cesarean was required because the baby's life was in grave danger.

It is a difficult matter, but the mother's health and the baby's health must be weighed against each other sometimes and a compromise made. In those cases where the fetus is in jeopardy, amniocentesis for fetal lung maturity is often done. There is a calculated risk assessment at that point: Can we wait until the lungs are ready and the baby can be safely delivered? Or do we accept prematurity and deliver rather than risk the fetus dying undelivered, or the mother succumbing to her severe disease? Giving the mother a type of potent cortisone called dexamethasone or betamethasone will speed up fetal lung development. When a baby is born premature, its lungs are not fully developed and need time to adjust to breathing air since they are underwater in the womb. If the breathing problem is severe it is called respiratory distress syndrome (RDS). RDS can be fatal if prolonged and severe enough. Giving dexamethasone to the mother allows it to cross into the fetus and stimulate rapid lung development over two or three days. After that time, it is effective and the fetal lungs will be developed.

That two to three days is a very tense wait. We pray that the baby will stay with us for those next two days until we can deliver it and that the mother's condition will not get worse. We want to give the baby the best chance for survival outside the mother, but prevent its death while still inside the mother—a tricky tightrope walk that we must do in these situations. We monitor mother and baby continuously, 24 hours a day for those two days, ready for an emergency Cesarean section to be done at a minute's notice. This is maximum intensive care: two patients, one inside the other, with both lives on the line. That is truly high-risk pregnancy. Obstetricians do it day in and day out with dedication to both patients—the mother and the infant. And the constantly improving technology of contemporary medicine is making it possible for us to save mothers who might never have lived through pregnancy and to save babies who might never have been born.

# fifteen

## ENDOCRINE CAUSES OF MISCARRIAGE: YES, IT'S HORMONAL

~~~~~~~~~~~~~~~~~~~~~~~~~~~~~~~~~~~~~~~~~~~~~~

## DENISE

WHEN I FIRST MET DENISE I ASKED HER TO TELL ME about her problem, an open-ended way to begin a medical interview. Denise told me her story from the start in detail. For their first wedding anniversary, Denise, just 26, and her husband, Sal, 28, went through the motions of honoring the occasion: an extravagant dinner at the restaurant where Sal had proposed, the ceremonial eating of the saved and de-frosted cake top from their wedding reception; an exchange of heartfelt gifts. But they were sad because the one gift they wanted for each other, a baby, was conspicuously absent from the celebration, she explained.

They were both in great health. Denise worked out regularly at her gym, and Sal, a telephone company repairman, had the kind of job that kept him on the move constantly. He even played in a softball league with some friends from work on the weekends. They were eager to start a family and spent that first 365-plus days of their marriage without using birth control. Then, as Denise started to question their fertility, she became pregnant. They were thrilled, she told me.

The minute Denise saw the positive results on her home pregnancy test, she phoned her doctor to make an appointment. She had scheduled a visit eight weeks from the date of her last menstrual period. Denise could hardly wait, she said. She began reading pregnancy magazines and checking out charted, interactive pregnancy calendars on the Internet. She said time took on that slow, engrossing sensation similar to being tucked into a movie theater, deeply involved in the story unfolding in front of your eyes. But it was their story—hers, Sal's, and the new family they were creating.

When Denise began bleeding and cramping, she called her doctor. The physician wasn't encouraging. Denise's doctor had logged 20 years in the ob/gyn field, and Denise felt confident and trusting of her medical opinion. The doctor said she believed that there was no intervention that would make a difference. She told Denise that if it was a normal pregnancy it would hold and she would stay pregnant; if it was not normal, she would lose it and would be better off that way. Denise was taken aback by this kind of hands-in-the-air approach. She asked that doctor if there wasn't anything that could be done. A test? Medication? Bed rest? Should she stop exercising? The doctor told Denise that she didn't believe that there was any treatment for a threatened abortion (a term that shocked Denise until the doctor explained that it was the medical term for a miscarriage) and that even bed rest wouldn't matter. Only time would tell.

After two weeks of anxiety, Denise lost the pregnancy in the tenth week and had a D&C performed by her doctor. This also proved to be a bit of a shock to Denise. She'd never had general anesthesia before, and had no idea what to expect. She quickly lost consciousness in the operating room, and she described awakening in another room, frightened and shivering from the cold sensation left over by the anesthesia. Sal was there waiting, watching Denise go from slightly bewildered to remembering where she was and why she was there. She began to cry as soon as she focused in on his face and the look in his eyes; she said, "He was looking at me so sadly."

In the follow-up appointment, Denise's doctor had offered encouragement and advised her to try again as soon as she felt up to it, adding that miscarriage was very common and not to worry about it. But the thing was, she was worried about it, and she was starting to feel she wasn't being heard by her doctor, Denise said, who didn't seem particularly open to Denise and Sal's questions and concerns.

When Denise came to see me for that first visit she had all sorts of questions that had not been answered. "Why did it happen to me? Did I do something wrong? I work as a cosmetologist using skin creams and hair dyes on my clients. Could that have made me lose my baby?" I calmed her as I answered all her questions.

I took a careful medical history from Denise, which is always the first step in diagnosis. In fact, about 80 percent of the diagnosis is in what the patient tells you. Denise was very good with details, and she told me some very important pieces of information: (1) her periods were becoming less regular, (2) she was not sleeping well, and (3) she was getting nervous and jittery. All of these clues made me think about a thyroid problem, and so I asked her more-specific questions about symptoms associated with that problem—and she had them:

1. *Sensitivity to heat.* Denise did not tolerate warm weather anymore even though she had always preferred it to cold.
2. *Extreme perspiration.* She sweated a lot even when not exercising, and when she worked out she could feel her heart pounding away in her chest.
3. *Change in bowel movements.* Her bowels were often loose.
4. *Change in appetite.* She always felt hungry and was eating a great deal more than she ever had but she was losing weight.

These were all symptoms of an overactive thyroid gland, a known cause of miscarriage. Not only that, but these symptoms often become more severe after a pregnancy or a miscarriage, and that was exactly what was happening to Denise.

Her physical examination provided even more evidence of an

overactive thyroid. Her pulse beat was fast. Her blood pressure was a bit high, and she appeared to be somewhat flushed. She was also slightly shaky, almost trembling when she held out her hands. However, I noticed something else during her exam that concerned me even more. There was a round, firm one-centimeter knot in her neck in the right lobe of her thyroid gland. This could not be due to swelling from a pregnancy. I ordered a number of further tests and recommended a thyroid specialist for Denise to see. The tests confirmed the presence of **hyperthyroidism,** but a biopsy showed that the knot in her neck was a cancer of the thyroid. Denise and Sal were stunned—this was, of course, the last thing the healthy young couple expected to hear.

---

### hyperthyroidism
The medical term for an overactive thyroid.

---

## OVERCOMING THE PROBLEM

Denise was devastated, and of course all pregnancy plans were canceled. Fortunately, though, thyroid cancers tend to be slow growing and spread only in the later stages of the disease. Denise's thyroid cancer was detected early and would be curable by surgery.

She had complete removal of her thyroid gland and was given thyroid hormone replacement. Her symptoms were gone and her menstruation became more normal. There was one complication from the surgery, though, that would require constant monitoring for the rest of Denise's life. The surgeon did not want to risk leaving any cancer behind and so removed the parathyroid glands, four small structures next to the thyroid. These small structures control your body's calcium. They produce parathyroid hormone, which regulates the absorption and storage of calcium in your body for strong bones and teeth, in conjunction with vitamin D and other hormones. Without these little glands, you would get osteoporosis (thinned-out bones) and lose your teeth. Denise would need extra calcium and vitamin D from now on to carry out the function of the now-missing parathyroid glands.

Two years after her treatment, Denise's doctors told her that she was cured. She and Sal were beyond relieved, even though they said she would have to be watched closely for many years to come. But then came the icing on the cake: not only was now 29-year-old Denise in remission, she was in the clear to try to have a baby again.

Denise arrived in my office soon thereafter to tell me the great news and to get started. I reviewed her laboratory tests from her thyroid doctors and they were all normal. I started her on prenatal vitamins. Also, even though she was undergoing replacement therapy for her calcium and vitamin D deficiencies since the removal of the parathyroid glands, I prescribed extra doses of both because she needed to take the extra vitamins and extra calcium, especially the extra vitamin D. An underactive parathyroid gland, just like an underactive thyroid gland, can cause miscarriages, too.

Four months later Denise had missed her period. Her periods had been slightly irregular and had become heavier over the years, so when she missed her period this time, she wasn't immediately convinced there was reason to believe it was a pregnancy. She hoped it was and had made an appointment to see me in two weeks, just in case. At two weeks overdue for her period, Denise phoned me to say that she'd started bleeding but wasn't experiencing any cramping. Over the telephone, I advised her to go home immediately from work and rest in bed and then to see me the next day. She could get her blood tests, her ultrasound, and her examination all in the morning.

The next day her examination and ultrasound showed no fetus in the uterus. Her blood tests showed that she had been pregnant, though, but it was over. It was too late to save it now. Even though Denise didn't realize she'd been pregnant until we ran tests, she was still shocked and upset. And who could blame her, after all she'd been through? What we needed to know now was why. The reason this time was too little thyroid hormone.

The blood tests revealed that her hormone levels were not enough to maintain a pregnancy. The thyroid-stimulating hormone was very high, but her thyroxine and triiodothyronine were just below the lower limit of normal. Her thyroid replacement requirements had increased during the previous four months and becoming pregnant had increased the need far beyond what she had been taking. In addition, Denise informed me that she had just run out of her thyroid hormone over the last couple of weeks and had not hurried to get more, since she was expecting to see me in two weeks.

I realized that Denise did not understand the full importance of remaining on her medication, so I explained that the problem of insufficient thyroid hormone could cause a miscarriage. Denise hadn't realized how much more she had to worry about. Further into the conversation, she began blaming herself for the miscarriage. I reassured her: the problem could be corrected by increasing her hormone dose and monitoring her blood tests every one to two months. Denise looked unsure but nodded. "Okay," she said, "I can do this, but I think I also need some time to recover. Emotionally, I mean—this second one really took us by surprise. And after the cancer...I guess we had a little more invested in this pregnancy than we even knew." I assured her that that made perfect sense and that she not only needed to be physically ready to try again, but giving herself time to heal from the emotional blow was important, too.

I did not perform a D&C because the entire miscarriage was over and complete with no visible tissue in her uterus on sonogram. I advised Denise to wait three menstrual cycles before attempting pregnancy again while we monitored her new dose of thyroid hormone every month. When she became pregnant again, we would continue this close monitoring until the third month of pregnancy. After that her blood would be drawn to check the dose every six weeks until delivery. This was important not only to assure staying pregnant, but to avoid hypothyroidism in the infant, a very serious condition causing mental retardation if not prevented.

All the tests were normal when Denise and Sal came back to see me for pre-conceptional counseling two months after the miscarriage. I could see there was still grief in Denise's eyes. Sal was wearing his telephone company repairman belt with tools attached over his jeans and red and black flannel shirt. He had left work early and come directly to our appointment, and I could see that this added to the tension he was already feeling. The corners of his eyes and mouth were creased with the telltale lines of stress, and as the couple sat in the two chairs across from my desk, Sal's right leg jiggled nervously. Both Denise and Sal were worried about entering into this for a third time and coming up empty again.

I gave Denise a starter supply of prenatal vitamins and extra calcium along with prescriptions for them and outlined a program for blood tests throughout the pregnancy. I explained, again, the importance of taking her medications and close follow-up. Finally, I told them I thought they were ready to try for the next pregnancy if they felt up to it, and that a normal pregnancy was well within the realm of possibility if they stayed with the program. Despite his nervousness, Sal said he was ready to give it another go. Denise looked at him for a moment and gave him a tiny smile. She then looked at me, exhaled, and said, "Then I guess we're all ready."

Denise meant what she said: she missed her next period and the hopeful couple was on their way. Denise took her medications faithfully and followed to a T the monitoring program for the next nine months. Between keeping a close eye on Denise and working overtime to prepare for the baby, Sal seemed to be the more frazzled of the two. Denise amazed both of us by remaining utterly calm. She seemed to be soothed by a schedule that she could stick to, knowing that it would keep her baby safe and make everything go as planned. The sonograms and blood tests were done on schedule, and I only had to increase the dose of thyroid

**hormone** once to meet the greater need of pregnancy. The baby grew normally and the pregnancy progressed very well.

Denise went into labor three days before her due date. She had a normal labor, epidural anesthesia, and a normal birth. Sal, of course, was there for the whole thing. As you'd imagine, the joy on their faces when they held their new son, Gary, was an incredibly rewarding moment. Afterward, Sal said that watching his $8^{1}/_{2}$ lb son being born was the greatest experience of his life.

---

## hormones

Chemical messengers produced by special cells in your body's organs. These organs are called glands. The hormones are released into your blood and regulate specific targets like your ovaries, blood vessels, kidneys, and other structures throughout the body.

---

## WHAT CAUSES HORMONAL PROBLEMS IN PREGNANCY?

Denise's problem with her thyroid hormone is just one of many different kinds of hormonal disease. All of your hormones have to be working correctly for a pregnancy to go forward normally. The thyroid gland produces two thyroid hormones, which control your **metabolism**. If the thyroid is overactive or underactive you may be infertile, you may miscarry, or you may have serious complications in pregnancy.

---

## metabolism

The chemical processes by which your body uses the food you eat as fuel to drive all of the body's functions.

---

The pituitary is the main gland that regulates the other glands. Think of it as kind of a mainframe computer, overseeing a network of other machines and sending out messages that help each of the individual network computers to do their job. The pituitary gland releases hormones that control these other glands, which include the thyroid and adrenal, and other organs. It also regulates the ovaries (and testes in men), breasts and lactation, contractions of the uterus, and kidney function. When there is a history of fertility problems or pregnancy loss, hormones should be evaluated by the appropriate blood tests. The table below shows the major hormones and some of their key functions.

## ENDOCRINE GLAND SYMPTOMS

| GLAND | OVERACTIVE | UNDERACTIVE |
|---|---|---|
| Pituitary | Diabetes, high blood pressure, obesity, large size, weakness, hair growth, irregular periods | Dwarfism, fatigue, low blood pressure, low blood sugar, sterility |
| Thyroid | Irregular periods, jitteriness, shakiness, increased appetite, weight loss, frequent bowel movements, heat intolerance | Infrequent periods, fatigue, decreased appetite, weight gain, water retention, constipation, cold intolerance |
| Adrenal | Diabetes, high blood pressure, obesity, hair growth, infrequent periods | Weakness, weight loss, low blood pressure, hair loss, absent periods, poor tolerance for stress |
| Parathyroid | Bone loss, abnormal calcified tissues, kidney stones, tooth loss, high calcium levels in blood | Bone loss, dental problems, poor growth, low calcium levels in blood |

The great news is that modern medicine can diagnose and successfully treat all of the hormonal diseases that may lead to miscarriage. Even in a patient like Denise, with cancer of the thyroid and complete removal of the thyroid and parathyroid glands, we can supply the missing hormones and maintain normal function.

In Denise's case, I closely followed her progress by tracking her specific hormone deficiency throughout her pregnancy via her blood levels. This is how we follow the levels of the specific hormones in question for any woman with hormonal problems because pregnancy will change the normal values for most hormones. So, for example, the two thyroid hormones (thyroxine and triiodothyronine) and the pituitary hormone (thyroid-stimulating hormone) are examples that are more complicated to follow during pregnancy because there are very specific changes in their normal values. The parathyroid hormone can be measured as well as calcium levels and these also are changed in pregnancy. In fact pregnancy affects all your hormones, and they may affect the pregnancy.

If you have a diagnosed hormonal condition, your doctor needs to know how to follow these changes in pregnant patients, and that there are differences in the hormone values from those seen in non-pregnant women. The thyroid and the ovary are the most common causes for pregnancy loss, but all of the hormone-producing glands can be trouble.

Whatever the hormone problem, the first step in treatment in order to sustain pregnancy is to replace what is missing or suppress what is overactive. After that, close monitoring of the hormone levels through blood tests with awareness of the normal values in pregnant women versus non-pregnant women is essential, as I did with Denise. Finally, ultrasound monitoring of the fetus at regular intervals and watching closely for possible complications in labor like high blood pressure are part of the care of not only these patients but all pregnant women. With skillful care, women with hormonal diseases can expect the same results as any other expecting mother.

# sixteen

## DIABETES: IT'S ABOUT CONTROL

~~~~~~~~~~~~~~~~~~~~~~~~~~~~~~~~~~~~~~~~~~~~~~~~~~~~~~~

## NANCY

IT BEGAN WHEN SHE WAS ONLY FIVE YEARS OLD. NANCY was very sick. She was thirsty all the time, constantly asking for water and going to the bathroom every hour. She ate voraciously but was thin and losing weight. And she smelled like nail polish. Her mom and dad were very frightened and brought their daughter to the pediatrician immediately to find out what was wrong. The pediatrician tested her urine and it was loaded with sugar and ketones, the source of the nail polish odor. She had obvious juvenile diabetes and needed immediate treatment with insulin.

Nancy's parents were actually very relieved to know what was wrong with her, they told her later on when she was an adult. They knew what was wrong with their daughter, how to control the disease, and could help her cope with it as a child. Now, 23 years later, Nancy sat in my office telling me her story and presenting me with her new challenge—she wanted to have a baby. At our first meeting, Nancy, now 28, recounted her history with diabetes for me. She'd been on insulin for 23 years, and had just lost her first pregnancy. She and her husband, Rick, wanted a baby very much and assumed that her insulin treatment, loosely followed after all these years, was just fine. Even though Rick was a urologist, they were both nonchalant about her diabetic control. After all, it had been under control for the last 20 years! And she usually followed her insulin schedule. Nevertheless, at eight weeks she had lost the baby and had a D&C.

Nancy was a short, thin woman with large brown eyes and light brown hair who had a softness about her that immediately made you feel like protecting her. She told me that she had been raised to be meticulous about her diet and exercise, and particularly her insulin. She also said that she was raised to be self-reliant and independent in spite of her diabetes. I know that what she said was true—after all, she was here on her own for this first meeting with no one holding her hand, and she spoke about her work as a psychologist and her great passion for helping people. Her manner, on the other hand, told me that she had always been protected by her family because her vulnerability was not shielded by a tough veneer, it was right out there for anyone to see.

Three years ago, Nancy married Rick while he was in his last year of residency training as a urologist. Now that he was out of training and in practice, they were ready to start a family. With this first pregnancy not working out the way they'd hoped, Nancy didn't want to risk another miscarriage or put her health in jeopardy by trying again without the help of a specialist. She was eager to try again, but worried about what might happen. She was also certain that this first miscarriage was her fault.

Rick was very supportive, and being a doctor made it easier for him to understand her needs as a person suffering with diabetes, and gave her the security of knowing that her partner knew as much about her disease and how to control it as she did. The term used to describe her diabetes was "brittle"—difficult to control. Nancy had long been on a complicated schedule of insulin injections that she had to give herself five times a day. In addition to that, she had to check her blood sugar at least five times a day, getting the blood via finger punctures. And while her kidneys and her heart were still undamaged by her diabetes, her eyes had been affected by the disease and had required laser retinal surgery.

## OVERCOMING THE PROBLEM

Nancy showed me her blood sugar results from the diary she had
to keep for recording them. They varied far too much for proper
control pre-pregnancy. Her menstrual periods were irregular, and
when I did a workup on her it showed that she also had irregular
ovulation. With this in mind, I knew that our plan needed to be
twofold: first, we needed to better control her diabetes, and second, I needed to improve the regularity of her ovulation. I referred
her to a new diabetes specialist who started her on an insulin
pump, a device that was integral in keeping tight control of her
blood sugar and that she could wear on a belt around her waist,
attached by a tubing to a fine needle inserted under the skin of her
abdomen. After two months of vigorous control and a month of
prenatal vitamins, I treated her with the ovulation-inducing drug
clomiphene. She was pregnant in the first cycle on treatment.

Her hormones progressed normally. Her blood sugar was kept
in the low-normal range by adjusting the dose of insulin continuously by means of the pump. As the pregnancy progressed, Nancy's
insulin need increased as it usually does with diabetes when all is
proceeding well. The baby grew normally, which was a great relief
to Nancy, whose first pregnancy ended at two months. Still, pregnancy for a diabetic is a tricky situation, and even after the first
three months there is a greater risk of pregnancy loss, so close
monitoring was necessary. Nancy not only had to check her finger-
stick blood sugars six times a day, she had to see the doctor every
two weeks, follow a specific diet, pay constant attention to her insulin pump, and go through many sonograms and nonstress tests,
because the baby could be lost at any time in pregnancy.

Depending on the severity of the diabetes, early delivery may
be required—and that was the situation for Nancy. I induced labor
at two weeks before her due date. After 12 hours of labor there was
no progress, and so Nancy agreed to a Cesarean section. Prolonged
labor increases the potential for worsening the diabetic condition,
and possibly overstresses an already stressed baby. I delivered a

very frisky boy weighing 6 lb 12 oz—mother and baby were fine. Two years later we repeated the performance for an adorable little girl. Nancy tried once more, at age 34, with less control of her diabetes because she had been lulled into complacency about her illness, and unfortunately she miscarried. With two healthy, happy kids at home, Nancy decided against another try after that. Neither child has diabetes and, in fact, both are very athletic and physically thriving. Nancy knows that exercise is a wonderful preventive measure for potential diabetes, and she and Rick love getting out for bike rides in the park with their kids. Today, thanks to her good habits and proper monitoring, she is a busy suburban mom, practicing part-time as a therapist and leading a normal life, save for the insulin pump and eyeglasses. For Nancy, diabetes had always been a normal part of her life from the time she was a child. Today, being a family is, too.

## WHAT CAUSES DIABETES?

Diabetes is the disease that is becoming rapidly widespread more than any other and affects millions of Americans today. Diabetes affects the way the body uses food. It is caused by a lack of insulin, a hormone made in the pancreas that is essential for converting energy from food. Insulin is necessary for the body to process nutrients (carbohydrates, fats, and proteins), and its absence causes high sugar (glucose) levels in the blood. There is a genetic aspect, but inheritance is complex, and just because a parent has it doesn't mean you will.

Type 2 diabetes affects older adults and rarely requires insulin. People affected by type 2 diabetes can usually control the disease with good diet and exercise habits, and sometimes oral medication. The other, type 1, affects all ages, even infants, and does require insulin throughout a person's lifetime. Type 1 diabetes is very serious and, if not treated properly, people will die. The good news is that we are able to treat type 1 diabetes patients and prevent early death and serious complications for almost all type 1 diabetics.

Because untreated diabetes can affect the eyes, the kidneys, the heart, and blood vessels throughout your whole body, it can cause many serious problems, such as with Nancy's vision and pregnancy loss. Miscarriage is just one of those problems, but it can occur at any time in pregnant diabetics, even at full term. Since we know that, every woman is routinely tested for diabetes at least once during a pregnancy because pregnancy will bring out diabetes in an undiagnosed patient and the risks are there even if the diabetes is mild. Not every woman is at risk because only someone who has the genetic program for getting diabetes can have it develop during pregnancy. Sometimes it recedes after the birth only to return later in life, and sometimes it persists.

## WHAT CAN BE DONE

Because of the continuing risk of fetal loss for a pregnant diabetic, close follow-up and intensive care are vital for these truly high-risk pregnancies. Tight control of blood sugar, as in Nancy's instance, is maintained. This is accomplished with the pregnant woman taking her own blood measurements by sticking her finger six to eight times a day for readings on home blood-glucose monitors. In addition, monthly sonograms are done and, in the last two months of pregnancy, weekly or twice-weekly fetal well-being is monitored. This is accomplished by performing **biophysical profile** testing and **umbilical artery Doppler blood flow** studies.

---

### biophysical profile
A combination of ultrasound and fetal heart rate monitoring to evaluate the fetal heartbeat, breathing, and body movements, as well as the amount of amniotic fluid present. If there is too little amniotic fluid, the risk of losing the baby is greater.

## umbilical artery doppler blood flow

A test using an ultrasound machine to evaluate the blood flow in the fetal umbilical artery in order to determine if it is getting enough blood flow through the placenta.

Finally, tests for fetal lung development may be part of a diabetic mother-to-be's prescribed monitoring to decide whether or not early delivery is necessary in the more severe cases. An amniocentesis may be done to obtain amniotic fluid for testing for **L/S ratio** or other tests of fetal lung maturity. If lung maturity is confirmed the fetus can be delivered safely.

## l/s ratio

A test done on amniotic fluid in which the chemicals lecithin and sphingomyelin are measured, and the ratio of the lecithin (L) to the sphingomyelin (S) is calculated. When the fetal lungs are producing enough surfactant, a chemical that keeps them open, the lungs are believed to be mature. The L/S ratio is an indicator of how much surfactant is present in the fetus, since lecithin is a component of surfactant and sphingomyelin is usually present in a steady amount throughout pregnancy.

When the lungs are mature the baby will not have breathing difficulties even if it is delivered before its due date. As long as the fetal tests are normal, the delivery can be delayed until we know that the lungs are mature. With today's medical technology and full patient cooperation, a diabetic woman has the same chance for a healthy baby as anyone else. As you saw with my patient Nancy, it is vital to be active in your treatment by closely monitoring your blood, going for prescribed sonograms and fetal well-being tests, and eating right and doing the best things possible for your body. But just like Nancy, controlling your disease and becoming a mom while maintaining your own health is not just a "maybe," it's well within your grasp.

# seventeen

## INADEQUATE CORPUS LUTEUM: TIRED OVARIES

~~~~~~~~~~~~~~~~~~~~~~~~~~~~~~~~~~~~~~~~~~~~~~~~~~~~~~~

### SHU-YI

AS THEY ENTERED MY CONSULTING ROOM, BOTH SHU-YI and her husband, Wei, were glum faced and barely responsive to my greeting. We sat down at my desk across from each other; I smiling and they expressionless and stiff. To break the ice, I asked how they came to see me. Without even looking at each other, Wei began the explanation while Shu-Yi sat in stony silence, her anger palpable to me without her so much as breathing a word.

Wei explained that Shu-Yi was a PhD biochemist at New York University and obtained my name from a member of her department. He explained that she had miscarried three times in their three years of marriage.

"Shu-Yi is forty-one, and we're beginning to worry that we're running out of time," Wei said, staring at the photos in my office of my patients and their new babies.

"We really want a child before she is too..." Wei broke off, and looked down. Shu-Yi flinched slightly at the word that wasn't spoken and gave Wei a blistering look.

I asked Wei about his age, which he said was 45; and I asked what his work was. He told me that he was an administrator with a New York City agency. He volunteered that they were both well established career-wise and more than ready for parenthood, but it just wasn't happening. I looked at Shu-Yi, who up to this point had said nothing, but who began to look uncomfortable. I started paying

closer attention to her. The easiest way, of course, was to begin taking her history.

All her miscarriages, she said, were before the third month and
resulted in bleeding and cramps. She had a D&C after each of
them, but had only had chromosome studies to look for a genetically abnormal embryo after the last one. That study was negative,
and Wei and Shu-Yi were at a loss as to what could possibly be
causing the problem.

The pattern was the same: each pregnancy had gone well until
six weeks, and then Shu-Yi began bleeding. Sonograms showed a
normal fetal heartbeat at six weeks, which then disappeared at
about eight weeks in the first two pregnancies; seven weeks in the
last miscarriage. In that one, the chromosomes were tested and a
normal male fetus was diagnosed. When Shu-Yi gave me this final
piece of information, her voice began to take on an angry tone, and
understandably so: she was left with no answers, an even more
frustrating predicament for a scientist like herself who looks to
facts and data to solve problems.

She asked me why this happened to her, and how it was possible that she lost a normal boy. Her doctor had told her the first two
losses were probably not normal; that she could accept. But why
did she lose this one?

"What could have been missed?" she asked, her voice rising and
sounding angrier and angrier with each syllable she pronounced.

I told Shu-Yi that I understood that she was upset and angry,
but our goal at that moment was not to blame, but to find out the
answers to her questions and, most important, get to her real goal:
a healthy baby. Although this was what she wanted to hear, of
course, Shu-Yi wasn't ready to believe it—not yet, anyway. Taking
the rest of her history and performing a physical examination was
not easy. With her lingering feelings of anger and disappointment,
Shu-Yi only grudgingly cooperated. It was a big decision for her to
make another attempt at pregnancy.

"I can't take another disappointment," she said, shaking her head. I knew if she was here, in my office, though, that despite her angry exterior, Shu-Yi had hope, and I felt there might be good reason to feel that way. With the help of Wei, I was able to persuade her to go through a workup as a preliminary step to one more potential try at pregnancy. I told her that if we could find the reason for her miscarriage, we most likely could correct it. If she was strong enough to try again I was confident we would be able to get her what her heart desired. This appealed to the scientific side of her, and she agreed. Still, her knowledge that her age and her husband's age increased their risk of miscarriage—a factor that obviously cannot be corrected no matter how hard we try—weighed heavily on her mind.

## OVERCOMING THE PROBLEM

After a detailed medical history and examination, one fact stood out: her menstrual cycles had become somewhat irregular. Shu-Yi usually had two or three days of spotting or staining before her menstrual flow and the flow was lighter than it had been in previous years. She was worried about that, too, because she was afraid that it might be the beginning of menopause and her chances for a child were dwindling with every menstruation. With this in mind, I ordered blood tests to measure her estrogen and progesterone levels during the middle of the **luteal phase** of her cycle.

---

### luteal phase
The luteal phase is the 14 days from the time of ovulation to the beginning of menstruation.

---

I ordered the other usual tests for thyroid and prolactin blood levels just to be safe, but I was hot on the trail of an inadequate luteal phase. To confirm that diagnosis I took a biopsy from the lining of the uterus at the middle of the luteal phase, which confirmed a lack of sufficient hormones to support an early pregnancy. This diagnosis of luteal phase deficiency is due to an inadequate **corpus luteum** in the ovary. When there is an inadequate corpus luteum producing a luteal phase deficiency, there is usually not enough progesterone to maintain an early pregnancy. Estrogen levels, however, are often sufficient, although in rare cases they are below the necessary amount to support early pregnancy, as well.

> ## corpus luteum
> The corpus luteum is the part of the ovary that secretes the hormones that support early pregnancy after ovulation. When pregnancy does not occur and the hormone levels from the corpus luteum begin to fade, menstruation follows.

The good news is that a luteal phase deficiency can be treated by adding progesterone after ovulation or by stimulating ovulation with the drug clomiphene, and by adding progesterone in early pregnancy if necessary to supplement the other treatments. This was the process I prescribed for Shu-Yi. She remained skeptical, but was brave enough to try clomiphene to induce a stronger ovulation. I even detected some hope behind her skepticism when I told her she had a 10 percent chance of twins with this therapy. For the very first time, I saw her smile.

She agreed to begin clomiphene treatment and embark on one last attempt at motherhood. Shu-Yi conceived on the second cycle of treatment, but her progesterone level remained in the low-normal range during the first week of pregnancy. This fact made Shu-Yi continue the steely demeanor I'd witnessed that first day in my office. I knew it wasn't an uncommon reaction in many women who experience pregnancy loss. She was trying to protect herself from another disappointment, especially since I had to tell her that these low progesterone levels could also be a sign of an abnormal fetus.

She was only 6 weeks pregnant when I began Shu-Yi on **progesterone vaginal suppositories**. I followed her progress closely with blood tests and sonograms over the following week. All the results were satisfactory, and the blood tests were continued twice weekly and the ultrasound every two weeks until she was far enough along to have a **chorionic villus sampling** (CVS). Until that was performed, she would not count on a normal baby.

Her numbers continued to rise into the high-normal range, and a sonogram at 10 weeks showed one normal-appearing fetus with a normal fetal heartbeat. We were okay so far, but we weren't home free until the CVS came back normal. At 10½ weeks I performed a CVS. Shu-Yi and Wei spent the next seven days on pins and needles—they'd never made it this far along in pregnancy; and the longer it progressed, the more attached they both grew to the idea that they might really become parents this time around.

---

### progesterone suppositories

A suppository that is inserted vaginally. Once inside the vagina, it softens and releases progesterone into a mother's body. This is used when it is necessary to augment inadequate progesterone production, a hormone that must be present at certain levels during the first ten weeks in order to ensure the continuation of a pregnancy. Not all pharmacies have the capability to make them, so if they are prescribed for you, be sure to check with your regular pharmacy first. Otherwise, ask your doctor for a list of pharmacies that provide them.

---

One week later the report came back 46XX: a normal girl. Further tests confirmed the diagnosis of a normal pregnancy, and we settled down to monthly sonograms and an only slightly less tense six months.

---

## chorionic villus sampling (cvs)

A genetic test performed at 10 to 12 weeks of pregnancy, where a minuscule piece of the placenta is biopsied in order to detect abnormalities with a fetus early.

---

At one week past her due date, Shu-Yi was beside herself with worry and Wei was just about the same, despite all my tests being normal and all the reassurance I could give them. They couldn't take it any longer and wanted immediate delivery, a Cesarean section, as soon as possible. I explained that spontaneous labor would be easier for her, but I had to give in in part because she pleaded with me to give her baby to her before something bad happened. I agreed to induce labor since there was little to gain by waiting, and they were both distraught already. Sixteen hours later Gracie was born at 6 lb 12 oz, and nothing less than adorable. There weren't a lot of smiles during that long road to parenthood, but Shu-Yi and Wei have been smiling ever since.

## WHAT CAUSES INADEQUATE CORPUS LUTEUM?

In order to understand the problem of an inadequate corpus luteum we need to review the way a pregnancy develops. After ovulation, the egg that is released from the ovary meets the winning sperm in the fallopian tube and fertilization occurs. (See Chapter 1.) The ovary that released the egg now has another job: hormone production. It starts to make large amounts of progesterone, the key hormone to support pregnancy, from the cyst that produced the egg. This cyst is called the corpus luteum (which means "yellow body" in Latin, because the large amount of progesterone in the cells of the corpus luteum gives it a yellow color).

The corpus luteum also makes lots of estrogen, and both hormones are needed to support an early pregnancy. The corpus luteum is needed for the first ten weeks of pregnancy, until the embryo grows its placenta to a large enough size for it to make sufficient estrogen and progesterone on its own. After ten weeks of pregnancy the placenta is self-sustaining. As we saw in her story, Shu-Yi wasn't producing enough progesterone due to a luteal phase defect, and needed to have this hormone supplemented until the placenta could support itself.

While the placenta is growing it produces some estrogen and progesterone in its early stages, but not enough to maintain pregnancy. The placenta seems to know this, though, because it makes a hormone called human chorionic gonadotropin (HCG), which stimulates the corpus luteum to make more estrogen and progesterone in order to allow the placenta and the embryo to keep growing. This mutual feedback mechanism is crucial to get an early pregnancy past the initial eight to ten weeks. Only then can the placenta take over, and the ovary is no longer necessary.

Sometimes the corpus luteum lacks the **enzyme,** or has insufficient functioning cells, to make the necessary amount of hormone, which is usually progesterone. Very rarely, in addition to or other than a progesterone defect, there is an estrogen lack, as well. The insufficient amount of hormones causes a short luteal phase with bleeding less than 14 days after ovulation. If pregnancy occurs, the placenta will not grow as well and cannot make enough HCG to maintain the feedback mechanism. When this occurs there is bleeding, very often followed by miscarriage. In fact, about 20 percent of recurrent miscarriages are due to corpus luteum deficiency from an inadequate corpus luteum.

> enzyme
> A protein that acts to cause a chemical reaction to go forward quickly.

## WHAT CAN BE DONE?

The diagnosis can often be suspected from the following clues:

- A history of shortening menstrual cycles
- Decreasing menstrual flow
- Spotting during the luteal phase

Be sure you note any changes to your cycle and report them to your physician. That is an important part of detecting—and resolving—this issue. However, it can be caused by many hormonal disturbances (see Chapter 15) such as stress, frequent travel to different time zones, variations in light exposure, extreme changes in weight, being just post-puberty, just pre-menopause, or post-partum, and sometimes for just no apparent reason at all, though that is rare.

Blood tests in the luteal phase can tell us a lot. In addition, an endometrial biopsy showing a three-day lag in the development of the uterine lining after ovulation, which should be thickening during that point in the cycle, can also help in making a diagnosis.

Specific hormonal causes like thyroid disease can be treated and the inadequate corpus luteum will be corrected. When there is no specific cause, progesterone treatment in the luteal phase and early pregnancy may be enough, but sometimes it is necessary to stimulate ovulation in order to overcome an inadequate corpus luteum and correct the luteal phase deficiency. However, in addition to stimulating ovulation it is sometimes necessary to supplement with progesterone during the pregnancy, as well, in order to get the best outcome, as was the case for Shu-Yi and Wei. In older women, especially after 40, the ovary often may not have enough reserve despite clomid stimulation. It is sometimes a problem even in young women.

It was certainly difficult for Shu-Yi and Wei not only to endure the pregnancy losses they did, but to know that one of them was a normal, healthy fetus. It's incredibly difficult to make the decision to try again when no answers have been found. Potential parents will inevitably think, "Should we risk another disappointment?" I'm very glad Shu-Yi and Wei found the courage, because when the problem is a luteal phase defect, there is nearly always a successful treatment.

# eighteen

## BLIGHTED OVUM: A BAD START

~~~~~~~~~~~~~~~~~~~~~~~~~~~~~~~~~~~~~~~~~~~~~~~~

## RUTHIE

RUTHIE LOOKED OLDER THAN THE 38 SHE SAID SHE WAS. Although she was a 14-year veteran of the New York City public school system, I would soon learn that it wasn't her job as a first-grade school teacher in Brooklyn that was wearing on her. I was standing in the doorway to my consulting room, waiting to greet her and her husband, Avi, a gregarious 45-year-old New York City cabdriver who emigrated to the U.S. years ago from Israel. As they walked down the hall to meet me, they held hands in the genuine, loving way that some couples do; the ones who you can immediately see draw strength from each other, going through life's joys and tragedies side by side as partners through the best and worst of it all.

For Ruthie and Avi the joy was their five-year-old son, Jake. When she spoke about him, the lines on Ruthie's face softened and Avi broke into a broad, proud smile. They loved their role as parents; so much so that after Jake was born they tried again immediately for another baby. Although she became pregnant within a quick couple of months, it ended in miscarriage by the eighth week. Upset, of course, but not put off by a long shot, Ruthie and Avi tried again. And again. Each of the subsequent pregnancies following the birth of Jake ended in pregnancy loss. And now, Ruthie was pregnant for the fourth time.

As she sat in my office, Ruthie explained that she had missed her period and was bleeding. Her regular doctor had not been able to see her, and, understandably, she was beginning to panic, so when she called, I squeezed her into my schedule.

Her history revealed no specific medical problems, and her family history was significant only in that her mother had maturity-onset diabetes. Avi said that his family was healthy, and there were no miscarriages or abnormal children on his side, either. Ruthie's physical examination showed that her uterus was enlarged to about six-weeks-pregnancy size, consistent with the date of her last menstrual period. There was a small amount of blood oozing from the opening of her **cervix**.

---

### cervix

The part of the uterus that protrudes into the top of the vagina and has an opening into the uterus. It is often referred to as the mouth of the womb.

---

A vaginal sonogram enabled me to confirm that there was a pregnancy in her uterus with no ectopic pregnancy, something I was concerned could be an issue. (See Chapter 11.) Early bleeding is often the first sign of a pregnancy outside of the uterus, in the fallopian tube. But although a fetus was indeed present, I could not detect a heartbeat. There was no reason to panic just yet: at this point in pregnancy that could be normal. Given her previous miscarriages, though, I was concerned.

I explained to Ruthie and Avi that this could be normal, but due to her history and the small amount of blood coming from her cervix, it was clear to me that I should treat this as a threatened miscarriage, and I explained that I would need further tests, and the information from her previous pregnancies, as well.

Ruthie's pregnancy history was complicated: one normal birth, an early miscarriage, a miscarriage at 16 weeks of pregnancy, and then another early miscarriage. There was no consistent pattern. I ordered a panel of tests for Ruthie to try to get to the cause of her problem. After that visit, she had her blood drawn to measure levels of:

- Progesterone, the pregnancy hormone supporting the lining of the uterus
- Estrogen, the major female hormone that increases with a healthy fetus and placenta
- Beta HCG, the major pregnancy hormone that is made by the placenta and increases in the first trimester of normal pregnancy
- Thyroid-stimulating hormone, which evaluates thyroid function
- Antiphospholipid antibodies, which can be high with recurrent abortion
- Antinuclear antibodies, seen with auto-immune disease
- Rheumatoid factor, seen with auto-immune disease
- Blood coagulation tests, sometimes a cause of miscarriage when there is too much or too little blood clotting
- A complete blood count, which evaluates for infection and anemia
- A platelet count, which can be low in many diseases and can cause bleeding if too low
- Full chemistries to determine the body's chemical balance, which can lead to miscarriage if abnormal

I requested her records from her previous pregnancies. I started Ruthie on **progesterone suppositories,** which she was to begin at bedtime that evening after the blood was drawn for testing. The test would show any hormonal deficiency, but treatment before taking the blood could mask that. I recommended that she stay home from work and rest until the bleeding stopped, and avoid sexual intercourse.

Since most miscarriages are due to an abnormal embryo (a **blighted ovum**), many doctors do not advise these steps. There is considerable controversy over these measures because there is not enough medical literature to support their necessity in the presence of a threatened miscarriage. If the pregnancy is abnormal these measures will not help the mother to hold on to the pregnancy, and we do not want them to. We do not want them to delay the process of miscarriage. However, if the threatened miscarriage is due to inadequate hormones, these tests will identify the deficiency and hormone therapy can save an otherwise normal pregnancy.

---

### blighted ovum

An outdated and often inaccurate term used to describe an abnormal ovum, or egg, as cause for an unhealthy pregnancy instead of an abnormal embryo as cause for miscarriage.

---

In addition, I believe that for the 20 to 40 percent of patients whose bleeding is not due to abnormalities of the embryo, and therefore not a blighted ovum, it is worthwhile to try to improve blood flow to the uterus by limiting activity. At worst, bed rest will not harm and not help. And in Ruthie's case, it did prove helpful because she stopped bleeding the next day, allowing us to get out of crisis mode and focus on monitoring her hormone levels. Her blood tests were normal, except for her progesterone level, which was low, and her beta HCG level, which was quite high, at the upper limit of normal. The beta HCG is produced exclusively by the placenta and can be very high when there is a chromosomal abnormality with extra chromosomes, especially with a **molar pregnancy**.

## molar pregnancy

The placenta is abnormal with excessive growth leading to hy-datidiform mole. There is no fetus or rarely there is a fetus present, but molar pregnancy always results in a miscarriage. Hydatidiform mole occurs about 1 in 2,000 pregnancies and can go on to choriocarcinoma, a type of cancer, in about 1 per-cent of molar pregnancies.

## OVERCOMING THE PROBLEM

Ruthie's son, Jake, was a totally normal five-year-old boy. Her records indicated an eight-week miscarriage and no D&C (dilation and curettage) with her second pregnancy, a sixteen-week miscar-riage with a D&C but no report of an abnormal fetus, and a six-week miscarriage with a D&C and chromosome studies showing an abnormal embryo with trisomy 18 (an extra chromosome 18), a condition that is not compatible with survival beyond the newborn stage and usually ends in miscarriage. Ruth's follow-up blood tests, after her first series with me, showed a rising beta HCG, but no in-crease in her progesterone level, an ominous sign.

Over the next two weeks, the embryo did not grow, the proges-terone stayed at the same level, and the beta HCG dropped by 50 percent. There was no bleeding, but this embryo had not survived. I performed a D&C, and the chromosome studies showed a triploidy, a chromosomal abnormality where there are one and a half times the normal chromosomes, an amount not compatible with life.

Ruthie quickly recovered physically from her D&C. At her six-week postoperative visit, I explained the problem to her, Avi, and little Jake, who came along since they could not get a babysitter. It was easy to see why Ruthie and Avi were eager to have another child and willing to take so many chances. Jake was a sweet, adorable little boy, very well behaved for a five-year-old. He sat quietly munching on a pretzel that his father had supplied for the visit and looking at the photos of moms and dads and babies that I keep on the shelf next to my desk. I explained to Ruthie and Avi that the miscarriage was unavoidable because the fetus could not survive even in the protected environment of the womb. It was not the same abnormality as the previous miscarriages and was un- likely to happen again. However, I needed to further evaluate Ruthie with more testing to try to discover the reason for her other miscarriages before they tried again.

After a full evaluation, which included a hysteroscopy, lapa- roscopy (each surgeries to evaluate the reproductive organs), and semen analysis, there were no abnormal findings. I explained that according to the follow-up tests and Ruthie and Avi's medical his- tories, all was well. The miscarriages were from unrelated, ab- normal embryonic causes. Lightning had struck this couple four times—it was either bad luck or something that we could not diag- nose or treat.

Because Avi was 45 and Ruthie 38, I explained to the couple that the risk of another miscarriage was at least one in three; oth- erwise there was no medical reason to discourage another preg- nancy try. By now, Jake and I were good friends, and he asked me for a brother. "It might be a sister," I told him. He looked at me, thinking over this new idea, and nodded his head: "Well . . . okay. But a brother is better." Jake's declaration made his parents laugh, and he smiled at them, pleased to have caused this eruption of cheer when moments before everyone had looked so very serious. With that, the decision had been made.

Ruthie and Avi did try again, and she conceived six months later. I followed the blood HCG, estradiol, and progesterone every three days as soon as the pregnancy test was positive. The numbers kept going up normally, as did the tentative hopes of Ruthie and Avi. The first two sonograms were normal with a good fetal heartbeat at 8 weeks. When the 10-week sonogram showed good growth of the fetus and a normal fetal heart beating very clearly, both parents had tears in their eyes. The next step was an **amniocentesis** done at 15 weeks and 4 days pregnant. The result was 46XX—a normal girl. Another month went by. Although hopeful with all the good news they'd received so far, the couple could still not fully believe that it was truly a normal pregnancy. At five months, Ruthie felt the baby moving, and for the first time since Jake was born she felt that she was going to have a baby.

---

### amniocentesis

A procedure through which a long needle is passed into the pregnant uterus through the mother's abdomen and a sample of the fluid around the baby is drawn off to be tested. Chromosomes and many illnesses can be looked for as well as fetal lung maturity. For Ruthie and Avi, chromosomes were crucial to verify a normal baby.

---

Mothers and babies can sometimes do the unexpected, so we obstetricians have to be alert to any sign of potential trouble. Even though all signs pointed to a normal, healthy pregnancy and there were no problems, I watched Ruthie and her soon-to-be-born daughter very closely. So, when my measurement of the size of Ruthie's uterus was less than expected at six weeks short of the due date, I performed a sonogram to check the baby's growth. It showed that the baby was indeed growing, but at the lower limit of normal progress compared with the previous sonograms. This raised a red flag and when I explained it to Ruthie very gently, she became alarmed. I tried to calm her by outlining my more intensive surveillance of fetal well-being. I ordered weekly **nonstress testing,** as well as a **biophysical profile** to evaluate the fetus's condition because of the slowed growth.

## nonstress test

A fetal heart rate test to evaluate fetal well-being by observing increases in the fetal heart rate associated with fetal movements.

## biophysical profile

A combination of ultrasound and fetal heart rate monitoring to evaluate the fetal heartbeat, breathing, and body movements, as well as the amount of amniotic fluid present. If there is too little amniotic fluid, the risk of losing the baby is greater.

The biophysical profile was satisfactory, but the fetus was not growing very much. The placenta was starting to fail. Ruthie, Avi, and I discussed the need for early delivery, as soon as the baby's lungs were mature. Without mature lungs respiratory distress would occur and the baby would need care in an intensive care unit. I performed another biophysical profile on the fetus a week later in order to closely track its growth. This time, the results showed a decrease in amniotic fluid levels to less than normal, and the baby definitely was not growing at all. I performed an amniocentesis this time to test for fetal lung maturity.

Three different tests were done on the fluid to check lung development and only two of them showed that the baby's lungs were ready to work properly once delivered. Ruthie and Avi were very worried, but they remained calm once they understood my concerns and my findings. To lose this baby at this point was not going to happen if I could help it. The biophysical profile test did not assure me that this baby would be safe inside Ruthie for another week; but these profiles cannot indicate the exact risk, just that one exists. After discussing the situation with Ruthie and Avi, they said, "Doctor, we trust you. Do what you think is best," putting the full weight squarely on my shoulders. I chose delivery.

At 37 weeks pregnant, the odds favor the newborn, and I could not accurately state the risks for the life of the fetus if it stayed inside Ruthie. I induced labor early the next morning. It went quickly and well. Ten hours later, with Avi by his wife's side and with epidural anesthesia so that Ruthie could participate fully in the birth, I delivered a 5 lb, 6 oz little girl, Emily. She came out crying even before her body was delivered—there was no doubt that her lungs worked just fine.

## WHAT CAUSES THE PROBLEM?
The term "blighted ovum" really should not be used any longer because it is not an abnormal ovum, or egg, that causes miscarriage, but an abnormal embryo, which is destined not to survive. Today, we know that the majority of spontaneous abortions (or miscarriages, in ordinary language) are due to genetic abnormalities in the conceptus. The egg may be defective, or blighted, but so could be the sperm that fertilized the egg. Either one or both may be the source of the **genes** that cause the embryo to die.

The genes are located on the chromosomes inside the nucleus of a cell, and humans have 46 chromosomes, which carry all the information that determines who you are and how your body works. Each egg and each sperm carry half the normal number of chromosomes—23. When they unite (fertilization) an individual embryo is formed and grows into a fetus, and then at birth it continues with its growth and development always controlled by the original DNA packages on its chromosomes. When there are two X chromosomes present, you are female, and if there is only one X and one Y, you are male. All the other chromosomes are the same for men and women.

> ### gene
> The specific package of DNA on a chromosome that directs a cell to make a specific protein.

Most of the defects that are easily detected are chromosomal defects. The process of making an egg or sperm sometimes can lead to minor defects in chromosome arrangement, as the eggs or sperm (germ cells) are formed. If one chromosome fails to divide equally and is lost in the process, there is one chromosome missing (monosomy), and that will cause an abnormal embryo. An example is Turner's syndrome, which is 45X, missing chromosome 46, which is the other X. Most of these embryos do not survive, but some do. In this instance, the resulting baby is always female. They may turn out to be short females who are sterile, but are otherwise normal, or they may have major heart defects and disabilities.

An embryo may have an extra chromosome because one fails to separate from the others and lags behind in the process as the germ cells are formed (trisomy). An example is Down syndrome with an extra chromosome 21 with three rather than two of the number 21 chromosomes. The result is usually miscarriage, but survival occurs sometimes, as well. The survivor can be a child with some mental retardation but otherwise normal, or may have serious heart and other defects in addition. These individuals can be male or female. There are also abnormalities in the total number of chromosomes; so, an individual may have three sets, one and a half times normal (triploidy, as with Ruthie's fourth pregnancy), or four sets, double the normal number, called tetraploidy. Such individuals cannot survive fetal life. Finally, there are numerous gene defects that can be detected by special techniques when looked for specifically, like sickle cell anemia or cystic fibrosis. These are inherited diseases programmed by genes.

Making it even more complicated, there are people who have the normal amount of chromosomal material, but their chromosomes are not arranged normally. These people are normal and they have what is called a balanced translocation, meaning that pieces of two different chromosomes have moved to the wrong place on different chromosomes from usual and exchanged places with each other. This is one of the issues that has caused my co-author Amy to miscarry. When germ cells are formed in these normal people, too much or too little genetic material can result. If one of these genetically abnormal germ cells forms an embryo, miscarriage is likely depending on how and where the imbalance occurs. Any person with the balanced translocation is called a carrier and has an increased risk for miscarriage even though their partner is normal. The risk of miscarriage is 25 to 50 percent, and the risk for having a baby born with unbalanced translocation is 1 to 15 percent.

## WHAT CAN BE DONE

The products of a miscarriage should be studied for abnormal chromosomes. Any couple with two or more miscarriages should be seen by a genetics counselor and consider genetics testing. Genetic testing can be done before pregnancy to assess risks that a couple may have. Age of 35 or more for women and 40 or more for men increases miscarriage risk. Such patients or those with a known family history of an inherited disease or a birth defect can be screened and may need prenatal diagnosis. In some cases, in vitro fertilization with preimplantation genetic diagnosis may be needed (see Chapter 6) in order to ensure that the embryo(s) implanted into the mother are free of the genetic issues at hand. Others may choose **chorionic villus sampling,** or they may elect to have amniocentesis at 15 to 22 weeks to assure that a normal fetus is present.

> ### chorionic villus sampling
> A genetic test performed at 10 to 12 weeks of pregnancy where a minuscule piece of the placenta is biopsied in order to detect abnormalities with a fetus early on.

For most patients, an abnormal embryo is not likely to be repeated if neither parent has abnormal chromosomes or is a carrier. The increased odds through age alone still offers a nearly two out of three (or at worst, a one out of two) chance for a normal baby. When miscarriages recur, but not with the same bad chromosomes, the chance for a happy outcome in the next pregnancy is the same as if there never was a miscarriage, like Ruthie and Avi. While this (understandably) is frustrating for those who want answers and who have endured several bad turns of the proverbial wheel of fortune, the main thing to understand and recognize is that having a normal, healthy pregnancy and a normal, healthy baby is still three out of four—a very good possibility for most couples.

# nineteen

## AUTO-IMMUNE DISEASE:
## WHEN THE BODY FIGHTS ITSELF

~~~~~~~~~~~~~~~~~~~~~~~~~~~~~~~~~~~~~~~~~~~~~~~~~

## DONNA

WHEN I MET DONNA AND HER HUSBAND, VINCENT, EVERY-thing about them appeared completely in sync. They sat down at the same time; grabbed for each other's hand at the same time. They had roamed the globe experiencing new places together, and that day in my office they both noted the photos of destinations I've visited on my office walls, having made the same trips themselves, among many others. By their third anniversary they knew that kids were the next step in their great adventure together. They were both only 29—time was on their side, and it seemed like the world was, too, Donna said.

When Donna miscarried twice within the first year—both pregnancies stopping short at the three-month mark—she and Vincent were collectively shocked, but they dealt with it in the same calm, centered way they handled everything together. They were apprehensive about trying a third time, sure; but they knew they were each young and healthy. There must be a reason for the problem and, hopefully, an answer to their odd misfortune. They were right.

Their doctor suggested that before trying again, the couple go see a specialist, which is how they came to sit across from me in my office at NYU Medical Center. As I began to question Donna about her medical history, I noticed that Vincent paid close attention, listening carefully to both what was being asked and the answers I received. Good thing, too—that quality turned out to be more than just a charming aspect of his personality; it helped me to pinpoint what was causing Donna's pregnancy loss.

## OVERCOMING THE PROBLEM

Donna's physical examination and blood tests revealed nothing unusual—she was healthy, menstruated regularly, and, while her mother had an underactive thyroid problem and her maternal grandmother had diabetes, my tests revealed that Donna's thyroid was normal. Her father and sister were healthy as well, and no one had repeated miscarriages in her family. Looking for other clues, I asked more questions, trying to get to the bottom of the mystery, but she continued to shake her head no to each of my queries about possible medical problems. That's when Vincent remembered the missing link.

"Excuse me, Dr. Young," he said, "but there was one thing that happened just before we got married that was unusual..." His sentence trailed off, and before he continued, Vincent turned to look at his wife.

At first, Donna's brow knitted into a question mark, wondering what her husband was getting at—and then her face changed. I could see whatever it was, she remembered now, too.

Vincent then continued with the story: "Donna gave blood at our local blood drive right before we got married, and she tested positive for syphilis."

"But I wasn't positive!" she said, waving her hands and laughing self-consciously. "It was a *false*-positive."

Vincent reached over and squeezed her hand. Donna smiled, exhaled, and went on with her story. She'd been pretty upset about the test results at the time, knowing there was no way she could have contracted syphilis. In fact, at first she didn't believe the test results and was furious! Donna's regular physician assured her it was likely an error, although when he repeated the test it came back positive again. In the end, Donna had to undergo a special test to prove that she'd never contracted syphilis.

Vincent laughed and said, "Oh, I wasn't worried about her anyway," as Donna rolled her eyes at him. But what they didn't realize was that this pre-marital goof-up was the clue I needed to focus on a specific diagnosis. Patients who have immune conditions where the body reacts against itself will often show up with a false-positive blood test for syphilis. This may be the only finding in a seemingly well patient with **auto-immune disease**—until she becomes pregnant and miscarries.

---

### auto-immune disease

The body's immune system is hardwired to create antibodies to fight off foreign invaders that enter the body and threaten to upset the status quo. Normally, this is a good thing—your own personal army defending you against attackers. Sometimes, however, the immune system misinterprets good cells as foreign entities, attacking them and causing ailments resulting from that fight. In the case of auto-immune disease and pregnancy, the mother's and the fetus's immune systems are communicating with each other and the mother creates antibodies against her own cells. These antibodies get into the placenta (afterbirth), which is the organ that supports and protects the growing fetus, and can affect the placenta and the fetus to cause damage and miscarriage. The placenta and fetus share certain cell markers (antigens) with the mother, and these are attacked by maternal auto-antibodies. The disease that makes your own body attack itself makes a pregnant woman's immune system attack the similar markers on the placenta and fetus, half of which come from the mother and half from the father.

Donna's diagnostic evaluation proved that she was one of those patients. Now I knew the cause of her miscarriages: her blood test showed that she tested positive for antibodies that were markers for **antiphospholipid syndrome,** an immune condition that made her body react against the fetus. In Donna's case, there was great news. Treatment for antiphospholipid syndrome is often very successful, and sometimes even downright easy—the problem can be resolved during pregnancy by using aspirin alone or, in some cases, aspirin and heparin, a blood thinner. When properly diagnosed and treated, the majority of patients will have their baby at or near full term.

---

### antiphospholipid syndrome
An auto-immune condition in which antiphospholipid antibodies are markers of disease in which a patient's immune system attacks her own cells and will attack cells in her placenta and fetus.

---

I started Donna on one baby aspirin a day before she and Vincent began to try for another pregnancy. Her antiphospholipid antibodies were fine and she became pregnant. Her hormone levels progressed normally, and a sonogram at 8 weeks showed a normal pregnancy with a normal fetal heartbeat. When Donna and Vincent looked at the sonogram's monitor, I could see the look on their faces that I know all too well—great hope mixed with equal amounts of apprehension. I watched her antibody levels with monthly blood tests, and the aspirin kept them down.

After a tense pregnancy of aspirin therapy and close attention, which included blood tests, sonograms, and quite a bit of worry, I stopped the daily aspirin treatment at week 37 of Donna's pregnancy because that is as safe as a full-term pregnancy. Donna and Vincent's generally calm demeanor was put to the test. For the three days Donna was off the baby aspirin, it was impossible for them not to feel tense, even though they'd made it this far. On the third day, I induced labor and, after 12 hours, Matthew Vincent arrived at 6 lb 8 oz. And, to everyone's great relief and joy, he was in perfect health. I'll never forget what Donna said to me as she held Matty in her arms, his tiny body swaddled in a blanket, a blue-trimmed bonnet covering his shock of dark hair, just like his dad's: "Baby aspirin is the right name for a pill that can get you a baby!" Clearly, she and Vincent were feeling more like their old selves again, plus one.

## WHAT CAUSES AUTO-IMMUNE DISEASE?

The cause of auto-immune disease is the mother's immune system reacting against her own cells in a hostile way to destroy them as it mistakes them for an invader. In pregnancy the mother's confused immune system recognizes similarities between the placental and fetal cells and itself, since they are half Mom's and half Dad's genes. So the confused maternal immune system attacks not only itself, but the fetus and placenta as well. There are several auto-immune diseases that you need to be tested for if you have the presence of antiphospholipid antibodies in your blood, which I will discuss later on in this chapter. Antiphospholipid syndrome is often a marker of auto-immune-related miscarriage, and sometimes foretells the arrival of a serious disease.

## ANTIPHOSPHOLIPID SYNDROME

Any woman with unexplained pregnancy loss after the first three months or repeated miscarriages should be tested for antiphospholipid antibodies. Just like Donna, between 5 and 20 percent of women with repeated miscarriages will test positive for the antiphospholipid antibodies. While men also get it, approximately 70 percent of people who do test positive for them are women.

Having antiphospholipid antibodies does not necessarily mean that you carry any auto-immune diseases because these antibodies may be present in the absence of any disease at all. However, when the tests are positive, it's extremely important for your doctor to perform a careful medical evaluation in order to look for several auto-immune diseases, such as lupus, rheumatoid arthritis, dermatomyositis, Sjögren's syndrome, and systemic sclerosis.

Even though you may be in the clear for an auto-immune disease, the presence of the antibodies can still be associated with problems such as miscarriage, as in Donna's case. In fact, the antibodies may be there without having caused any trouble in your life at all, until many years later when you experience a miscarriage or, in some instances, develop an auto-immune disease.

The antiphospholipid antibodies most often present, called **anticardiolipin antibodies,** will cause a false-positive test for syphilis, just like they did for Donna. Most likely, the antibodies are not causing disease but are marking the existence of a reaction by your body against some of its own components. About half of such patients have another disease like systemic lupus erythematosus, while the other half have only the syndrome. But a condition that causes miscarriage is disease enough.

---

### anticardiolipin antibodies
A form of phospholipid antibody that resembles a component used in a standard blood test for syphilis.

---

However, there are other concerns when antiphospholipid antibodies are detected. Besides early miscarriage, there may be repeated miscarriages and other pregnancy complications. Miscarriage may occur at any time from early on in pregnancy to the late third trimester; most often late first or second trimester with the antiphospholipid syndrome. If you have antiphospholipid antibodies, you are also at an increased risk for blood clots in your veins and arteries while on birth control pills or when pregnant.

While most patients have no symptoms until something brings them out such as pregnancy, birth control pills, or surgery—especially pelvic surgery—any challenges to the female body may make problems caused by antiphospholipid antibodies apparent for the first time. There are other serious problems that may arise besides miscarriage, too, and that should be considered as potential signals of antiphospholipid syndrome. Illness like stroke, deep-vein blood clots, skin problems like blanching of the fingertips and toes with occasional skin ulcerations of the fingertips (Raynaud's phenomenon), anemia, and pulmonary embolism (blood clots in the lungs) may occur as the first signs of the antiphospholipid syndrome.

The treatment for this syndrome is still being debated among physicians, but it generally requires an agent to lower the risk of increased clotting of your blood, like aspirin or heparin.

## OTHER AUTO-IMMUNE DISEASES

There are other auto-immune diseases that may need to be diagnosed and properly managed in order for a woman to have a successful pregnancy and in order for her to be in her best health throughout her life.

An example of an auto-immune disease that might be present and that has serious effects is **systemic lupus erythematosus,** which not only shows these antiphospholipid antibodies but will often have lupus anticoagulant, a circulating protein in the blood that, in spite of its name, causes increased clotting. These lupus anticoagulant antibodies give rise to abnormal blood clots in veins and arteries. They are not always present and are not part of the definition of lupus.

> ## systemic lupus erythematosus
> A generalized auto-immune disease that damages joints, skin,
> lungs, kidneys, and other organs.

There is another pregnancy-related immune disease, Rh allo-immunization, which is known to cause miscarriage and fetal death. First recognized 50 years ago, the basic problem with this condition is a difference in blood type between the fetus and the mother. Eighty-five percent of Americans are Rh positive. However, among the small percentage that are Rh negative, women who plan to become pregnant need to be aware of the serious issue created by an Rh negative mom carrying an Rh positive baby.

Think of Rh allo-immunization as biological xenophobia. When the fetus is positive for the **Rh factor** on its red blood cells but the mother is negative, the fetal red blood cells entering into the mother's bloodstream cause an immune reaction in the mother against the fetus's blood. Because of their contrary Rh markers, the mother's body sees the fetus's cells as foreign. The mother's body then produces antibodies, which cross the placenta into the fetus and destroy the fetal red blood cells as though they were invading bacteria. Why? The mother's immune system sees the fetal red blood cells with an Rh surface marker not on its own cells as foreign invaders, and thus kills them. When enough blood cells are killed, the fetus is left in a serious state of anemia. If the anemia is severe enough, the fetus will die.

> ## rh factor
> Everyone has a blood type—A, B, AB, or O—which can be pos-
> itive or negative. Your Rh factor is a marker (antigen) on your

red blood cells that is either positive or negative. While most people (85 percent) are Rh positive, a small percentage are Rh negative.

The culprit in 98 percent of the patients who are affected with this condition is Rh negative cells in the mother reacting against Rh positive cells in the fetus because of a specific fetal antigen (a molecule on the surface of a cell that can be recognized by the body's immune system). Capital D is the most common antigen, and others are C, c, E, and several more that are very rare. This reaction of one person's immune system against antigens from another person is called allo-immunization, and in some cases may cause second-trimester miscarriage.

While this might sound like a frightening form of self-inflicted biological warfare, these days it is highly preventable. About 20 years ago, medical research resulted in a vaccine to prevent it. Today, whenever an Rh negative woman has a miscarriage, she is now given an injection of Rh immunoglobulin vaccine, as well as during the course of her next normal pregnancy, and right after childbirth. This will prevent the disease from occurring in 99.9 percent of cases.

Although this is the most common form of blood incompatibility, there are other kinds that cannot be prevented by the Rh vaccine. However, these are very rare—they make up only 2 percent of blood incompatibility issues—and for them, as well as Rh disease, only after at least one pregnancy or miscarriage will this become a problem, and only after several pregnancies will it be severe enough to cause miscarriage. That is why when a patient has a history of recurrent second-trimester or late-first-trimester miscarriage, different blood group compatibility problems should be looked for to rule out blood incompatibility as the cause. These tests detect specific antibodies in a maternal blood sample, and can routinely be done in blood banks.

But let's get to the best news here: today, Rh disease is almost totally gone in the United States and Western Europe. Over a period of 50 years it was identified, studied, and a treatment—the Rh vaccine—developed, preventing it in virtually all potential cases.

## WHAT CAN BE DONE

If you have had recurrent miscarriage, or any of the problems I've mentioned in this chapter, we can make the diagnosis from your medical history, as well as from blood tests showing the abnormal antibodies. Be aware, though, that the blood tests alone are not enough, as up to 5 percent of normal women will test positive. Every positive test must be followed up with a second one, as it is estimated that of women with repeated miscarriages, 15 percent have the antiphospholipid antibodies. But just like Donna, these women can be treated successfully with baby aspirin before and during their pregnancy. Some may also need heparin therapy, especially if they have had problems with blood clotting.

The notion that your body could react against that of your growing fetus may well sound crazy. After all, how could a mom attack her own child? But the human body is an amazing creation, and with all the things that it does right, sometimes a function or two can go haywire. The thing to keep in mind, though, is this: with a 75 to 80 percent success rate in preventing miscarriage in women with auto-immune disease, there is more than just the hope of having a healthy pregnancy. The statistics are on your side. Still, we physicians look forward to the day that we can say that the antiphospholipid syndrome has been 100 percent prevented. With an 80 percent cure rate for preventing miscarriages from the antiphospholipid syndrome in most auto-immune conditions, and a 99 percent prevention of Rh disease, I think we're getting close.

# twenty

## BLOOD-CLOTTING DISORDERS: TOO MUCH OF A GOOD THING

~~~~~~~~~~~~~~~~~~~~~~~~~~~~~~~~~~~~~~~~~~~~~~~~~

## CAROL

DR. ELINOR GARNER WAS CALLING FROM GREENWICH, Connecticut, and needed to speak to me immediately, my receptionist said. I knew Elinor when she was one of our brightest medical students at New York University's medical school, and was pleased when she chose to specialize in obstetrics and gynecology. Her husband was working toward becoming a surgeon and training at a different but equally prestigious hospital. Elinor chose to undergo her specialty training at the same institution as her spouse so they would have the opportunity to grab a few moments together during their time-consuming residency programs. Over the next decade, Elinor kept me abreast of her career and called me for advice or a consultation when she needed it. Over the last seven years, she had established a thriving practice in Greenwich and on this day, she needed me to consult on a patient matter that concerned her greatly.

She told me that she had a patient who was bleeding on and off for the last four weeks and was only four months pregnant. Elinor had the patient admitted to the hospital and treated her by bed rest and a blood transfusion. The bleeding had stopped, and the patient had just been discharged from the hospital that day. Elinor wanted me to accept her patient for continued care because she felt this was too complicated for her practice. Her diagnosis was chronic abruptio placentae, which is a partial but continued tearing off of

the placenta resulting in bleeding, with each episode preventing healing of the previous tear. Her call was on a Monday and I
squeezed her patient into my Tuesday schedule.

The patient was a 32-year-old children's book author named
Carol. She appeared more like a down-to-earth and stylish professor than the way I imagined a children's book author would appear—her straight brown hair was cut pixie-short and she wore a
warm brown tweed suit with an orange scarf tied around her neck.
I was a little surprised at how calm and composed she was for a
woman who was pregnant and bleeding on and off for a month. It
seemed to me after we chatted about her hospitalization that there
was a strong denial effect causing her apparently unworried attitude.

Her husband, Arthur, had driven her from Connecticut to New
York for this visit and joined us for the initial interview and subsequent discussion. He was 37 years old, dressed in a charcoal-gray
suit appropriate to his position as an investment banker, and, in
contrast to Carol's calm, unruffled demeanor, he wore a serious expression, accenting the early crow's-feet that had developed at the
corners of his brown eyes. They had put off starting a family so
Carol could anchor her writing career and Arthur could make
some rain at his Wall Street firm. This was their first pregnancy
and Arthur, a man who clearly didn't like wild cards in his life, was
unsettled by the unexpected bleeding in this very early stage of
their first pregnancy.

After getting them settled in my office, I took Carol's medical
history, which was not particularly revealing. She had always been
healthy and so were the members of her immediate family.
Arthur's medical history revealed nothing that could be related, either. Carol's physical examination was normal, and a sonogram
showed an active 18-week fetus and a normal amount of amniotic
fluid around it. The placenta was in the appropriate spot at the top
of the uterus. What the sonogram revealed that did concern me
was a large blood clot between the placenta and the wall of the

uterus where it was attached. That type of blood clot is called a subchorionic hematoma and it confirmed Dr. Garner's diagnosis of chronic abruptio placentae. But was there some reason for it? I wondered. I knew that their problem could get worse unpredictably, but it could also get better without treatment, depending on the cause. If the cause was a **thrombophilia,** then I could treat her and preserve the pregnancy.

> ## thrombophilia
> A blood-clotting disorder in which there is a tendency to excessive blood clotting under certain circumstances.

After I explained the problem and answered their questions about causes and possible treatments, I had to leave them in an unsettled state of mind. I didn't know the reason for the placenta problem and would have to wait for answers. I sent Carol for some blood tests that afternoon and prescribed bed rest at home because too much activity could increase the risk of bleeding again. I told the couple that heavy bleeding could occur without warning and, if that happened, to call me immediately and come to the hospital directly. Carol's composure changed almost imperceptibly as she struggled to remain calm. By this point, they fully understood the gravity of Carol's condition and were ready to do what it took to keep the pregnancy and Carol's health safely intact.

Sure enough on Wednesday morning at five-thirty A.M. Arthur called; Carol was bleeding heavily and had severe abdominal pain. I told them to come in immediately. Arthur had driven furiously to the hospital. They had bypassed the admitting office at my instruction and came directly to the delivery suite. I was waiting for her at the hospital. When I finally saw her and Arthur an hour and a half after that call, Carol was bleeding furiously with large blood clots the size of golf balls. Her cervix was 5 cm dilated and the legs of the fetus were in her birth canal because her water had already broken. It was too late to save the fetus, but I was able to save the mother.

## OVERCOMING THE PROBLEM

That night, Carol stayed in the hospital. The following day, I sent her home with some medication to keep her from bleeding more. On Friday, her blood test results came in. She had a thrombophilia, factor V Leiden mutation. Factor V Leiden mutation is a genetic condition that predisposes a mother to abnormal clot formation in the placenta, which leads to pregnancy loss in many of the cases. Overwhelming as that may sound, Carol's type of thrombophilia was treatable. I explained this to Carol and Arthur over the phone that day. They wanted to know how likely it was that this could happen again, and the risk to Carol. Carol told me that she was shaken by her first experience, but the fact that her condition was treatable made her sure she wanted to try again. She was eager to hear what would need to be done to ensure a healthy pregnancy next time around. I advised Carol and Arthur to use condoms for birth control for two cycles until Carol was fully back to normal and her uterus restored to its normal condition. That way the post-pregnancy state of Carol's womb would be gone, and it would be in the pre-pregnancy mode. I also explained that the next pregnancy would require heparin treatment, once- or twice-daily injections of an anticoagulant, which would decrease blood clotting and prevent pregnancy loss in about 75 percent of cases.

Six months passed. I wondered how Carol and Arthur were doing. Then Carol called with good news: a missed period. I saw her that week and her sonogram confirmed a six-week viable fetus. I sent her for the standard tests and repeated her thrombophilia blood tests. Everything was normal, except for the existing factor V Leiden mutation.

Two weeks later, another sonogram showed a normal living

fetus, appropriately grown to eight-week size. I began her heparin therapy and showed her and Arthur how to do a **subcutaneous injection** at home. Twice-daily shots would be necessary for the next seven months with careful monitoring of the blood-clotting tests to be sure that we were using the correct dose. The couple was terrifically cooperative in every way: they did the shots religiously and came to New York City for blood tests and exams on schedule. Both of them maintained that facade of composure during an outwardly very normal pregnancy. If they were worried, they never showed it.

---

### subcutaneous injection

An injection that is shot into the body just below the dermal and epidermal layers of skin into the subcutis layer.

---

Finally, we got to 38 weeks of pregnancy and it was time to discuss bringing on labor because I had to control the timing to avoid complications in cases like Carol's. I had to stop the anticoagulant in order to avoid a hemorrhage with childbirth. That needed about 24 hours to wear off completely after all those months of treatment, and I wanted to have a controlled delivery with everything ready in case of an unexpected emergency. So, we scheduled an induction of labor for 38 weeks and 4 days, just 10 days short of full term. Carol was willing to have her labor without an epidural anesthesia, which held a very slight risk of bleeding into her spine due to her being anticoagulated earlier. Everything had gone so well up to this point that Carol opted not to take even the smallest risk. She had a totally natural childbirth with 10 hours of induced labor. At 6:42 P.M., I delivered a 6 lb 8 oz screamer—a healthy little girl. Little Audrey made so much noise that I jokingly predicted a career as an opera singer for her. Two days later, Carol, Audrey, and Arthur went home to get acquainted with each other at last.

## WHAT CAUSES THROMBOPHILIA?

Thrombophilia means "clot loving" in Greek, which is a good description for this condition. When a patient has thrombophilia, there is too much protection against hemorrhage because she does not need the extent of blood clotting that is present. This increased risk of blood clotting can occur under conditions like pregnancy, surgery, trauma, or taking birth control pills.

The other kinds of blood-clotting disorders are called hemophilias, meaning "blood loving" in Greek, and they are associated with increased risks of bleeding. The large majority of hemophilias (but not all) are either not associated with increased risk for pregnancy loss or are almost exclusively diseases of males. If you think about it, this makes perfect sense—with hemophilia, a woman would hemorrhage with puberty and the onset of menstruation. Women would be likely to die before they got around to reproducing, so the disease could not be inherited. On the other hand, increased blood clotting—thrombophilia—would protect against hemorrhage and so would be more likely to be passed on even though pregnancy loss might be increased.

Not all of the thrombophilias are associated with an increased risk of pregnancy loss. There is still quite a bit of controversy among doctors about which ones are, and to what degree they increase the risk. The medical literature has not been conclusive for the thrombophilias seen with auto-immune disease (see Chapter 19) or for the inherited thrombophilias, such as in Carol's case. It is generally agreed, though, that with some thrombophilias, a pregnancy will end by the first or second trimester. Why this occurs is still not agreed upon by doctors entirely, but it appears that increased blood clotting where the placenta attaches on the uterus causes that part of the placenta to lose its necessary blood supply and die. The attachment comes loose at that point, and the blood vessels that are still open bleed into the space where the dead part of the placenta was attached. If the bleeding keeps up, the placenta continues to loosen and further detach from the uterus like a loose tooth wiggling away from the gum line. This causes vaginal bleeding and, if most of the placenta tears off, the pregnancy is lost and the mother may hemorrhage in spite of the increased blood clotting.

## WHAT CAN BE DONE

In studies on fetal loss with thrombophilias, only the following thrombophilias were associated with pregnancy loss:

factor V Leiden mutation
prothrombin gene mutation 20210A
activated protein C resistance
protein S deficiency
lupus anticoagulant
antiphospholipid syndrome

Only three of these have been highly associated with miscarriage: the lupus anticoagulant, the antiphospholipid syndrome, and the factor V Leiden mutation are the ones reported in the most studies. Patients with miscarriage, especially recurrent miscarriage, should be evaluated with blood tests for these blood-clotting abnormalities, as well as for antiphospholipid antibodies and connective-tissue disease.

When they are positive for the thrombophilias, a woman with a single dose of the abnormal gene (heterozygous) is at a lower risk than someone with a double dose (homozygous), but the exact risks are still unknown. In fact, even in normal women who are not afflicted with thrombophilia, the risk of a serious blood clot or propagation of a blood clot to the lungs (embolism) is increased in pregnancy and post-partum. In thrombophilia patients, though, that risk is greatly increased, and in double-dose women it is up to ten times the risk in single-dose women.

So, the risk of miscarriage for a patient with thrombophilia is not the only problem. A blood clot problem with possible lung damage is a concern as well, and both of these issues require some form of "blood thinner," also called an anticoagulant. Most common is aspirin, either alone or in combination with heparin. When the patient has already had a miscarriage, either regular heparin or low molecular weight heparin, a long-acting form of heparin, is usually prescribed for thrombophilia patients. The treatment is usually begun after eight to ten weeks of pregnancy and supplemented with 4 to 5 mg doses of folic acid and sometimes aspirin, as well. Whenever there is a history of an episode of a blood clot in a vein or artery, stroke, or embolism in a patient or a patient's family, thrombophilia testing should be done by your doctor.

Because the genetics are not fully worked out and individuals vary greatly, doctors cannot predict from the blood tests the pregnancy outcomes or chance for a serious complication. It is frustrating and unfortunate that the exact risks for a woman with a thrombophilia gene are not known, either for pregnancy loss or for thrombosis (forming a blood clot) and embolism. Neither are the exact benefits and risks of therapy with aspirin, low molecular weight heparin, or regular heparin. Currently, low molecular weight heparin is the most commonly used because it is usually one injection daily. However, it is believed by most doctors that anticoagulant treatment is beneficial in preventing pregnancy loss in these patients in two-thirds to three-quarters of those treated. Your doctor will decide on the best management for you, not only during but also after pregnancy, when blood clots in veins are most often diagnosed. Diagnosis, as always, is most important because treatment is effective when we understand what we are treating and why.

# section four

~~~~~~~~~~~~~~~~~~~~~~~~~~~~~~~~~~~~~~~~~~~~~~~~~~~

ENVIRONMENTAL HAZARDS:
WHEN NATURE DOESN'T NURTURE

# twenty-one

## INFECTIONS: GERM INVADERS

~~~~~~~~~~~~~~~~~~~~~~~~~~~~~~~~~~~~~~~~~~~~~~~~~~~~~~~~~~~~

### MONICA

WHEN I FIRST MET MONICA SHE WAS 18, WITH BROWN
hair and striking yellowish-hazel eyes. She was wearing designer
jeans, a white T-shirt with ST. TROPEZ in blue across the front,
and an uncomfortable look on her face. She arrived for her appointment 20 minutes late, announced herself to my receptionist,
and stated that she did not want to be kept waiting. My receptionist politely explained that Monica's lateness might well further delay her appointment, to which the young, new patient responded
by folding her arms across her chest and narrowing her eyes. "Do
you *know* who my father is?" she almost snarled.

This was Monica ten years ago. And while her attitude certainly sounds awful, it was mostly a mask. Monica's doctor had
asked her to see me because of abdominal pain that came and
went, most often in association with her menses, but sometimes
not related to the onset of menstruation at all. She was a teenager
and she was scared. Her mom was being treated for a fast, aggres-
sive form of Hodgkin's lymphoma. Her father—a well-known cap-
tain of industry—was worried about his wife, busy with his
stressful job, and, besides, had no idea what to say to a teenage girl
experiencing severe pain during her period.

So there Monica sat, sullenly perched across from my desk, act-
ing a bit immature even for her young age. I remember how she
appeared at first, brushing invisible pieces of lint from her pressed

jeans, legs crossed, and sitting up perfectly straight. She was so closed in during our initial conversation. As I talked with her, taking her history slowly, Monica's mask dropped. "I don't understand why I feel this kind of pain. None of my friends have this!" The pitch of her voice grew as she became almost angry, saying the things that had been on her mind for some time that she had been unable to say to her dad. "Why do things happen to me?" she blurted. "And my mom keeps worrying about me and making me crazy." Then I understood she was covering up her fear of cancer, fed by her mother's illness and her father's distraction. I calmed her down and told her that I did not feel she had cancer, and continued taking her history. Her menstrual pattern was irregular, and she often had prolonged spotting or staining up to ten days. Her spotting sometimes came in mid-cycle, too. The symptoms didn't immediately point to anything particular, so I ran several tests after reviewing the information from her internist. I examined Monica, too, and still there weren't any answers as to why her cycle was irregular or where the pain came from.

With no other obvious answer, I decided to first attempt to regulate Monica's abnormal cycle with six months of progesterone hormone treatment. This helped; she was better, but not completely. The pain was better and manageable, but the abnormal bleeding persisted. At that point, I performed a laparoscopy and hysteroscopy in order to try to get a clear diagnosis. Monica had an asymmetrical uterine septum, a rare anatomical abnormality.

"An asymmetrical what? Is that dangerous?" she said when I gave her the news. Her mother came with her and I gave the facts to them both. Monica's uterus was divided into two unequal parts with a small channel between them just at the level of the connection between her cervix and the inside of her uterus. The result was an uneven shedding of the lining of her womb as each side broke down and was shed through the small opening at the cervix. This is what was causing her irregular menstruation. As for the pain she was experiencing, that was a result of the smaller side of her divided uterus becoming swollen due to the blood filling it. When the larger side contracted to expel its menstrual contents, she also had pain, and since they each were shedding at different rates, she had both irregular pain and prolonged irregular menstrual bleeding and spotting.

The progesterone had helped by thinning out the uterine lining. The septum was something caused by abnormal formation of her uterus during fetal life, I explained. Her mother exclaimed, "Did it come from something I took or did?" I asked her if she recalled taking DES (see Chapter 10), and she had not taken any drugs while pregnant with Monica. Happily, I was able not only to diagnose the problem through the use of hysteroscopy, I was also able to fix it. I had removed the dividing septum through the hysteroscope using tiny scissors and grasping forceps. After that, Monica's periods were just fine. But that was only the beginning of Monica's story.

Monica remained my patient over the years. Her stress declined as she achieved normal menstrual cycles and time passed. She grew into a capable, kind adult—a mature young woman to everyone who knew her, including my office staff. Eventually, Monica married Darin. They were both 24 and in the rising phase of their young careers. Monica was selling advertising space for a magazine, and Darin was working at a top consulting firm. Their ambitions kept them engrossed in their respective careers—and when they weren't working hard, they were taking adventurous vacations that always involved foreign travel. But after four years, they started to feel that tug; something felt like it was missing from their lives, and they knew it was a child. At 28 years old, both Monica and Darin knew it was time to start a family.

Monica was worried, though. Despite the fact that her menstruation had been completely normal since the procedure I'd done on her a decade before, Monica wanted to know if there was any likelihood that it could affect her fertility. She'd been doing lots of reading on the Internet about her previous condition, and she'd seen some instances where women had miscarried. Both she and Darin quizzed me extensively at their pre-conceptual visit, and I gave them the facts: the risks were slightly increased for miscarriage, but it was still not especially likely.

Monica looked apprehensive, and knowing both her physical and family history, I could understand why. As much as becoming a parent is a tremendous milestone for any adult, for Monica it was a way to address the mother/daughter relationship that complicated her own life when her mother became ill. Darin, too, seemed to pick up on his wife's worries, and spoke up: "Well, I'm an MBA, and the way I figure it, the percentages are in our favor. We'll wait and see, but I really do think there's very little reason for concern." He exuded reasonableness and calm from his dark-brown eyes, and it was clear to me that he was going to be a great source of strength for his wife.

Monica went off her birth control pill. A month later, she had not conceived and she was immediately worried. Over the phone one April afternoon, I tried to reassure her that one month was nothing to worry about and that if she didn't conceive within the next five months, then I'd have her come back in for some further testing. Worrying wasn't doing much for Monica's outlook, but she said, "Okay, Dr. Young. I trust you and I'll hang in there."

One month later, on an early spring afternoon in May, I got another phone call: Monica was pregnant. Her home test was positive—three different times.

All was going along well, until the sixth week when she developed a cold, which normally wouldn't be a concern but this one came with a slight fever. A sonogram at seven weeks showed a normal fetal heartbeat, but Monica's cold hadn't gone away and now she had a fever of 101 degrees. She had been at her parents' home in Connecticut, and called their internist because he was nearby and she could get to his office quickly. When she described her symptoms, he asked her to come in right away. He was worried about Lyme disease.

Connecticut deer were the original source of the debilitating disease, and Old Lyme, Connecticut, was where the disease was first identified due to an infection transmitted by deer ticks. The internist took blood tests and began her on antibiotics, giving the first dose by injection into her left buttock. She called me right after seeing him, very concerned about Lyme disease, taking these antibiotics that the internist had prescribed, and the fever that just wouldn't go away. She was right to worry about Lyme disease and fever causing miscarriage, but not about antibiotics. Some antibiotics may have fetal effects, like jaundice of the newborn with certain sulfa drugs, or deafness in children exposed to drugs like gentamicin, or abnormal teeth developing in children exposed to tetracycline during pregnancy, but the large majority of antibiotics have no relationship to miscarriage at all. She saw the doctor the next day for more blood tests and another injection. Then she began an oral antibiotic, as well.

The next week, Monica called me because she had redness, tenderness, and swelling at the site of one of her antibiotic injections and was still running a fever, although it remained between 100 and 101 most of the time. I advised her to put hot compresses on the site of the irritation, and come to see me the next day. When she came into my office, Monica's fears were realized.

I examined Monica and performed a sonogram. At eight and a half weeks, there was no fetal heart present, and the fetus had not grown past what was seen at her last visit. A miscarriage was inevitable. Monica stared at the black and white screen, focusing on the clearly visible but utterly still outline of the fetus she was carrying. She closed her eyes. Tears leaked slowly from under her clenched eyelids. She couldn't speak.

## OVERCOMING THE PROBLEM

Monica pulled herself together, got dressed, and met me back in my office to talk things over. I told her I would schedule a dilation and curettage for her within the next few days, and that we would examine the fetus to find out exactly what happened. After the D&C the fetus turned out to be a normal female, but there was evidence of infection in the placental tissue. The cultures from the conceptual tissue (embryo and placenta) were negative for the bacteria that most commonly cause Lyme disease and positive for the bacteria that are commonly present on the skin, which can cause serious infections sometimes. Unfortunately, Lyme disease cultures can be negative, even when the disease is present, and skin bacteria cultures can be positive even when they are not causing illness. As is often the case, even with modern medicine, the cause could have been either of these, or something not tested. One thing was certain: the miscarriage was caused by an infection.

After a full evaluation to exclude any chronic infection, immunosuppression (a weakened immune system), depressed immune state of a chronic illness, and diabetes, it was clear that none of these conditions existed. I encouraged Monica and Darin to try again and reassured them that it was very unlikely that a similar experience would occur. She was doubtful, her voice revealing that her self-assurance was gone. "Something always happens to me," she said plaintively. Darin took her hand and said, "We can do it. Next time for sure, Monica."

Five months later, Monica was pregnant again. Her hormone tests were normal, and she felt fine, not even having nausea. Of course, that worried her. "Why am I not sick to my stomach?" she asked me anxiously during an early visit. "I've read that the more nauseated you are, the stronger the pregnancy is. There must be something wrong!" I explained to her that presence or lack of nausea meant nothing specific. (See Chapter 7.) There was nothing wrong with not having nausea. Still, Monica's previous miscarriage put doubt in her mind and she worried it would happen again. Even her anxious parents spent the first three months of Monica's pregnancy in an overly cautious state, staying put in their Manhattan penthouse and steering clear of their Connecticut house. Nobody wanted to take any chances. Monica could not get away from believing that her problems were some kind of terrible fate that she couldn't avoid—first with her period, then her abnormal uterus, and then her miscarriage. She kept waiting fearfully for the next complication. Even Darin began to look less composed. He and Monica had begun to eat out of nervousness, and the sympathy pounds he gained were starting to keep up with Monica's.

At their visits, I kept on reassuring them. The pregnancy progressed normally. At each sonogram, I could see Monica and Darin holding their breath, afraid of what they'd see, or not see, on the screen. But each and every time, we all saw a normally progressing fetus, growing just as it should. When Monica went into labor on her exact due date, it was finally taken as a sign that fate had changed its mind and was at last smiling at Monica. In fact, the labor went so well, Monica joked later that maybe, just maybe, her luck had changed. Her lucky charm: 6 lb 14 oz Linda, who was born after ten hours of labor, her huge brown eyes squinting in the light as she wiggled and squawked in the delivery room. She was beautiful just like her mother at this moment. And as she held her daughter for the first time with Darin by her side, I knew the only fate at work here was that Monica finally got her wish. She was able to overcome the pain, the tricks of fate in her life, the sadness, all of it. She was a mother at last.

## WHAT CAUSES INFECTION DURING PREGNANCY?

Any infection severe enough to produce prolonged high fever—an oral temperature over 101 degrees—can be a cause of miscarriage. That does not mean that every high fever for one day, or even three or four days, will cause a spontaneous miscarriage every time. In fact, this happens only in rare cases. On the other hand, some infections will cause a pregnancy loss without noticeable symptoms or with just the mild symptoms of a cold. There are some infections that are suspected as causes of recurrent pregnancy loss, as well.

What are these infections? Some are bacterial, some are viral,

and some from other kinds of infectious agents. The bacteria that
are specifically associated are:

*Listeria* (listeriosis)
*Brucella* (brucellosis)
*Borrelia* (Lyme disease)
*Treponema pallidum* (syphilis)
*Streptococcus* and *Staphylococcus* (strep throat and skin sores)
*Vibrio comma* (cholera)*
*Salmonella* (severe diarrhea, vomiting)*
*Shigella* (severe diarrhea)*

There are also very, very rare organisms seldom seen in the developed world that are associated with pregnancy loss. In addition,
there are viral diseases that may cause pregnancy loss:

- Cytomegalovirus (CMV), which causes a mild respiratory
  illness in most patients and is barely noticed
- Parvovirus B19, which causes a mild upper respiratory in-
  fection in most patients
- Human immunodeficiency virus (HIV), which causes AIDS
- Varicella, which causes chicken pox
- Rubella, which causes German measles
- Herpes, when it is the first infection with herpes
- Coxsackie virus: although suspected, it has not been clearly
  shown. The Coxsackie viruses are associated with a variety
  of symptoms ranging from upper respiratory infection to
  abdominal distress and diarrhea.

Recent research has identified viral DNA in preterm labor and
pregnancy loss patients' amniotic fluid and in fetal tissues. It is not

*Cholera, *Salmonella*, and *Shigella* cause miscarriage in *very rare instances*.

clear to what degree such viruses may cause miscarriage, but much research is pursuing this direction.

Other agents thought to be involved in miscarriage are mycoplasma and ureaplasma, which have been implicated in recurrent miscarriage and preterm births, but not proven to be a cause of pregnancy loss. These organisms are like bacteria, but do not have the normal cell wall seen in bacteria, and the infections they produce are often completely without any symptoms.

Finally, there are organisms that are single-cell structures called protozoans, such as toxoplasma and malaria, which sometimes can cause miscarriage when there is an acute infection. There are other potential agents of infection with varying degrees of symptoms, or no symptoms at all. Although they can be difficult to diagnose because of their slippery, altering symptoms, there's also no need to lose sleep thinking about them. The infections listed above are the most common and best identified as associated with miscarriage.

## WHAT CAN BE DONE

Monica's miscarriage was associated with symptoms of an infection, so it was possible to obtain specific information about the cause. Cultures were taken in an attempt to find the culprit, but even with them, it could only be narrowed down and not identified as one specific cause. Finding the exact cause of an infection is helpful because prompt treatment can prevent miscarriage in many cases, but sometimes it can be difficult to pinpoint what the exact infection is.

We can look to some clues, however. If the miscarriages are recurrent, agents like listeria, syphilis, or toxoplasmosis may be the cause. The good news here is that these are rare, and they can be treated and the problem corrected. Usually, it is a severe acute infection of unknown source that will cause a miscarriage, and most often that infection is bacterial. Blood, urine, throat, and vaginal cultures, or vaginal smears for microscopy can help make the diagnosis. The key to dealing with bacterial infections is, of course, immediate treatment. If antibiotics are initiated promptly, they are most often completely effective. It is acute, primary viral infections that can be tricky. Herpes simplex can be treated to prevent miscarriage using drugs like acyclovir, but for most viral infections there is no satisfactory treatment. Only vaccination *before* the infection can be preventive, as in the case with rubella (German measles), an illness that can cause miscarriage or serious fetal damage even though maternal symptoms are mild and often missed because the telltale rash is present only briefly. Women with HIV, even without active AIDS, are at an increased risk for infections, and thus for miscarriage. So are women on chemotherapy or immunosuppressive drugs because of an organ transplant, like a donated kidney. Women on long-term steroids, like prednisone for diseases such as lupus, and diabetic women, as well, are also at increased risk for infections in pregnancy. In fact, pregnancy itself is an immune-suppressed state. That is why your system does not normally reject the fetus.

But before this starts to sound like the script to a nightmare, remember: in all likelihood, you were vaccinated for most common viral infections long before you were pregnant, and vaccination is almost 100 percent effective in preventing these outcomes. For other viral diseases, like hepatitis A and B, or influenza, vaccination before pregnancy is prudent. When you are gearing up for pregnancy, the best prescription is to plan ahead since it may take a while for immunity to develop. If you are pregnant and develop fever, a rash, burning during urination, sore throat, diarrhea, or have been eating raw meat or handling kitty litter, call your doctor.

The thing to keep in mind (and that will keep you breathing easy) is that despite the suppression of the mother's immune system, which occurs normally in pregnancy, she is usually able to resist infection enough to avoid a miscarriage. Sometimes, you need a little help from your physician friends, as well. The correct diagnosis by cultures and by DNA tests for the infecting agent makes that easier to accomplish and can prevent miscarriage. If a miscarriage happens, culturing and DNA testing of the tissue passed out of the womb can be helpful in deciding about treatment to prevent further problems. Unfortunately, sometimes this information is not obtained, often because the samples are not processed correctly or they have become contaminated, or often because they just were not tested.

Still, the great majority of miscarriages related to an infection are one-shot deals—they happen once and they never happen again. Unless a woman is suffering from an immune suppression over and above that which normally occurs during pregnancy, she will become much more resistant to an infecting agent that she has met before. If you have had toxoplasmosis, for example, another infection is usually resisted, even in pregnancy, and the fetus is protected by antibodies. For nearly all pregnant women, an infection can make you sick—it may even make you very sick—but very rarely will it make you lose your pregnancy.

# twenty-two

## TOXIC AGENTS: GREENING YOUR PREGNANCY

~~~~~~~~~~~~~~~~~~~~~~~~~~~~~~~~~~~~~~~~~~~~~~~~~~~~~~~~~~~~~~~~~~~

## SUSAN

SUSAN WAS A WOMAN WHO ALWAYS HAD THE WILL AND the competence to achieve her goals. She was a first-rate emergency room doctor and proud of it. If there was something she wanted to master, she did it; if there was a problem to overcome, she beat it. But there was one lingering achievement that, until we met, remained just out of her grasp.

Susan was referred to me by her husband, Jerry, who was a practicing internist at my hospital. Three years ago at the young age of 37, Susan was diagnosed with early stage II breast cancer. A physician herself, she detected the lump in her right breast while doing her monthly self-examination in the shower. Thinking that the lump could potentially be a benign cyst, she decided not to panic and waited a month, until after her next menstrual period. It was still there—the size and hardness of a tiny pebble.

Susan sat across from me in my office telling her story, and it was as if I were talking with any other colleague about a patient, she was so matter-of-fact. She showed no emotion at all as she related the details like the facts on a medical chart: the diagnosis from her breast doctor, the mastectomy, the three positive lymph nodes, and the chemotherapy afterward. It wasn't until we got to her reason for being in my office that her demeanor changed. Susan wanted a baby and it was not working, she said with a tight, anxious note in what I came to know as her usually steady tone. She told me that she had stopped menstruating during her chemotherapy, and while her menstrual period was back to normal now, it had come back very slowly after the treatment was finished. As a physician, she knew that chemo was highly toxic, so she followed her cancer doctor's advice, and waited two years after her last treatment before she began trying for pregnancy.

The month before she came to see me, she had miscarried the only pregnancy she had ever achieved. I could hear the disappointment in her voice as she related the experience to me; I understood immediately what was unspoken, her unhappiness, her feelings of why me?, and her profound sense of failure. Susan had accomplished so much professionally; she had even been able to overcome the cancer, but now she could not carry a baby.

I started at the beginning as I always do and took the rest of her medical history, which was unrevealing, except for her menstrual pattern. Her menstruation was always heavy, lasted six or seven days, and occurred at about 35-day intervals, with the exception of when she was taking oral birth control. She had gone off the pill four years ago in order to become pregnant—a plan that had been interrupted by the cancer. But she was back on track now and, true to her great spirit and strength, she told me that she was ready to try again. When she miscarried she began to lose her self-confidence. As she sat there with me in my office, I could hear the doubt creeping into her voice. Finally, she said it, her voice thickening as she held back her threatening tears: "I'm forty and I don't have much time left. Do you think it's the cancer?"

## OVERCOMING THE PROBLEM

The combination of her advanced age for childbearing and her previous cancer was beyond Susan's usual strength after she miscarried. "I worry that I could die before ever having a child," she said to me that day in my office. The miscarriage was not related to the cancer itself because the cancer was gone, and even advanced cancer seldom ends a pregnancy. But cancer survivors always fear that anything going wrong could be due to the return of their cancer. When I assured her in no uncertain terms that the pregnancy loss was not related to cancer, it was as if a tight band around her emotions had been released and the tears came. I placed a box of tissues on my desk in front of her and she grabbed a few, blotting her eyes and exhaling as if she'd been holding her breath for a long time—in a way, she had been.

The miscarriage was at six weeks of pregnancy, and Susan had not had a D&C, but her uterus was normal size when I examined her. Most of her examination proved normal as well, except for the scar on her chest where her right breast used to be and some scarring present in her right armpit where the lymph nodes had been removed. I also saw that, compared to her left side, there was a noticeable enlargement of her right hand and arm, a common condition post–lymph node surgery called **lymphedema**. She said that she was getting physical therapy when I asked her if she had treatment for the lymphedema, and she was on no drugs now. But this, too, would not affect her ability to hold a pregnancy. Despite the scars on her chest and armpit, there were other signs of the healing taking place in Susan's body: her shiny black hair had grown back, and she said that it was even thicker than before the chemo.

---

## lymphedema

The lymph system is in part responsible for "filtering" the fluid that surrounds your cells. With lymphedema, a buildup of fluid occurs in the lymphatic system, which causes swelling and discomfort and, at worst, greater susceptibility to infection. While there can be other causes of lymphedema, it is not uncommon in breast cancer patients who have had lymph nodes removed with the cancer as part of their treatment.

I explained to Susan that we had to wait until after her next menstruation to do a proper evaluation in order to schedule the test at the right point in her menstrual cycle, but I already had a suspicion about her problem.

As a physician, Susan knew a great deal about her own problem, but she was eager to hear what I thought and I told her: "Chemotherapy affects your eggs, probably reduces their numbers, and may even leave some damaged ones. Also, you are a late ovulator and already prone to **luteal phase deficiency**. [See Chapter 17.] I think we can confirm the diagnosis in your next cycle and rule out any other causes by doing a cycle day-three **FSH** and **estradiol,** and then doing a hysterosalpingogram and luteal phase blood test for estradiol and progesterone. Then, I will do an endometrial biopsy," I told her. "By two months from now, we can treat the problem if I'm right."

---

## luteal phase deficiency

The luteal phase is the 14 days from the time of ovulation to the beginning of menstruation. A lack of sufficient hormones to support an early pregnancy is a luteal phase deficiency. This happens when there is an inadequate corpus luteum producing an inadequate amount of progesterone.

---

## fsh

Follicle-stimulating hormone is secreted by the pituitary gland and causes the ovary to ripen eggs to be ovulated.

---

### estradiol
The major female hormone, an essential component of female physiology.

---

I was right. I began treatment with clomiphene, a drug to induce the pituitary gland to release FSH, to induce an ovulation earlier in the cycle in order to achieve a better luteal phase. After three cycles, Susan was again pregnant, but her ovary was not quite up to it, as her progesterone tests were not rising at six weeks of pregnancy. Anticipating this possibility, which occurs often in such cases, I had given Susan a prescription for progesterone vaginal suppositories. When I got the test results showing that her progesterone levels were not rising as they should, I phoned her to say that now she needed them. She was to take one every night until the tenth week of pregnancy, which was one month away. I explained that by then the placenta would be taking over and self-sustaining, and she could stop the medication. It worked perfectly.

The pregnancy progressed normally. An amniocentesis at 16 weeks told us that it was a normal boy. At 39 weeks and 3 days, labor began. Jerry helped Susan as her coach, and got almost as involved in the process as his wife, both of them getting red in the face from holding their breath and pushing with each contraction. Finally, after 14 hours, 7 lb 1 oz Max was born. He was beautiful, healthy, with lots of black hair just like his mom.

## HOW AND WHEN DO TOXIC AGENTS AFFECT PREGNANCY?
Toxic agents can be thought of in different categories and can be divided into the following:

- Infections
- Alcohol
- Smoking
- Drugs
- Medications
- Radiation
- Environmental toxins
- Food poisoning

## Infections

There are several infections known to cause miscarriage. These include brucellosis, syphilis, listeriosis, mycoplasmas, and viruses such as cytomegalovirus, parvovirus, rubella, and varicella, as well as the one-celled parasite toxoplasmosis, among others that are even less common in the United States. Specific tests can determine the cause of an infection. Brucellosis, syphilis, and listeriosis are bacterial infections known to cause miscarriage. Mycoplasmas are a type of bacteria that may be a cause but the evidence is inconclusive. The viruses and toxoplasmosis are organisms that have been proven to be able to cause pregnancy losses in some patients. However, any severe infection with fever and microbes in the bloodstream can cause miscarriage or fetal malformations. (See Chapter 21.) If you have fever, even without other things like vomiting or flu-like symptoms, call your doctor.

## Alcohol, Smoking, and Drugs

The most common agent of pregnancy loss and fetal injury in this country is probably alcohol, followed by smoking, and then illegal drugs.

ALCOHOL The under-grown fetus of alcohol abusers that is not lost will have malformations and neurologic damage proportional to the amount of drinking during pregnancy. However, we are not talking about one or two drinks during a pregnancy, but persistent drinking on a regular basis that will harm the fetus and may lead to pregnancy loss, or an abnormal baby with **fetal alcohol syndrome**.

> ## fetal alcohol syndrome
> The resulting birth defects caused by severe alcohol abuse by a pregnant mother, which include neurological abnormalities, growth retardation, developmental disabilities, and physical abnormalities.

SMOKING Smoking does not have a known syndrome like fetal alcohol syndrome, but we know for sure that it increases the miscarriage rate and produces babies that are small for their due-date size and who may later have health problems. The more smoke exposure to the fetus, the more it is affected. Like drinking alcohol, if it is continued, regular smoking throughout pregnancy causes a bad outcome, but not an occasional cigarette. However, concerns have been raised about secondhand smoking so that the partner of a pregnant woman may cause fetal harm by smoking himself. The data on this is not yet conclusive. When you think about the known problems due to smoking, it should make you toss out your pack for the sake of your baby's health, and your own.

DRUGS Drugs such as marijuana, heroin, and morphine-like drugs of various kinds can affect the user's chromosomes, and pregnant users have more miscarriages and abnormal babies. However, it is not possible to separate out the drug from the many other factors in the lives of these women who are users. They often endure poor general health and tooth decay, malnutrition and infection, abuse and poverty. Their addiction is not only dangerous to their babies, it is dangerous to themselves. The most worrisome are amphetamines (speed), crack, and cocaine addicts because they are prone to mid-pregnancy miscarriage due to an acute separation of the placenta. This is usually associated with severe maternal hemorrhage and very high blood pressure. These women may not only lose their babies, they may suffer heart attacks, strokes, and even lose their lives.

## Medications

Believe it or not, some of the most innocuous medicines, prescribed and unprescribed, can actually be dangerous to a fetus. There are many drugs whose effects are not known, and the Food and Drug Administration has a classification for drugs in pregnancy and breast-feeding:

- *Class A.* Drugs that are safe to be taken during pregnancy and breast-feeding.
- *Class B.* Drugs whose effects have not been fully evaluated in humans, but have not shown bad effects when studied in animals.
- *Class C.* Drugs that have not been adequately tested in humans, but have shown bad effects in pregnant mice or rabbits or any other animal.
- *Class X.* Drugs that are known to have bad effects, such as increased miscarriage or malformations in people. Examples of Class X drugs are thalidomide, formerly an antinausea drug; Accutane for acne; and methotrexate, a chemotherapy drug. Most of the chemotherapy drugs are class X and their effects may be long lasting or even cause permanent infertility.

There are other drugs and substances, however, in most of our medicine chests and often used that you might not have even thought about as risky or mentioned to your doctor. These include aspirin, vitamin A and D, and indomethacin (usually seen in Motrin or similar drugs). All of these, in excess, have been linked to greater risks of pregnancy loss.

Even more concerning are the things that people take without any medical basis. The various mixes of plant extracts, teas, and assorted special ingredients that make up the category of herbal remedies and therapies have never been tested or in many cases never even analyzed for the chemicals in them. The best they could be would be pregnancy category B, but the Food and Drug Administration exempts these agents from testing because they are sold as food additives, not medicines. You will notice this when you read the fine print on their labels. Also, combining different drugs and herbals may have serious effects, like the serotonin syndrome with high blood pressure, confusion, and muscle spasms. Taking certain anti-depression medicines along with antacids or even with certain hard cheeses with moldy rinds could cause that kind of reaction. Many patients who have these kinds of symptoms cannot be diagnosed because no one knows what the herbal remedies are that they have been taking. Even if the FDA doesn't consider them as medications, for the purposes of a healthy pregnancy, you should. If you don't know what's in it or how it can truly affect you and your baby, just don't take it.

## Radiation

Radiation is a hazard that is greatly exaggerated. (See Chapter 7.) Despite what you might have heard (or, possibly, even read), X-rays, CT scans, and dental X-rays are not enough radiation exposure to cause a miscarriage or malformation. The radiation from the TV will not harm you or your pregnancy. And while there has been much conversation about the risks from computer screens or cell phones, you are not putting yourself or your baby at risk if you work on a computer on a daily basis or talk on a cell phone. And while we're at it, being near an electrical line or power plant is not a risk for miscarriage, either. While there is very little experimental information about atomic power plant radiation or medical tracers with radioactivity for diagnosis, neither are likely causes of miscarriage, unless there is a reactor failure the likes of Chernobyl or radioactive iodine therapy for carcinoma of the thyroid administered during pregnancy. (See Chapter 4.) However, radioactive iodine will concentrate in the fetal thyroid gland, as well as in the mother's, so pregnancy is not the time for this treatment of thyroid cancer and thyroid surgery is preferred. Passing through the detectors at an airport security gate is not hazardous. Neither is putting your finger into a detector at Sesame Place to let you back in.

Magnetic resonance imaging in pregnancy has not been shown to have any harmful effects leading to miscarriage or malformation, so strong magnetic energy does not raise any worries. Neither does ultrasound imaging, which uses high-frequency sound waves and bounces them off the baby without any serious consequences detected in the 35 years that it has been used.

### Environmental Toxins

Exposure to chemicals in pregnancy is more common than we realize. Some are dangerous; many are not. Women who work in industries where they are exposed to chemicals such as benzene, formaldehyde, lead, mercury, or insecticides should try to avoid direct contact with these chemicals, by wearing gloves or by asking for a different job assignment.

Paint fumes and solvents, cleaning fluids, nail polish and hair treatments, household bleach, rubbing alcohol and ammonia, soaps and detergents, are everyday examples that we all encounter. Most paints today are now water-based and therefore safe to use if you are pregnant. Oil-based paint is not going to cause a miscarriage, even when the fumes give you a headache. Solvents and paint thinners are not implicated in miscarriage unless there is daily exposure and direct contact; simply smelling the fumes will not cause a miscarriage. Cleaning fluids like spot removers, rug cleaners, furniture polish, and topical antiseptics like rubbing alcohol or peroxide are not associated with miscarriage. Soaps, detergents, bleach, and ammonia, even with direct skin contact, are not causes of pregnancy loss. Nail polish and the polish remover are not harmful to pregnant women or their fetuses.

Hair treatments, including coloring, curling, bleaching, and straightening, are often treated with caution in pregnancy. A wide variety of chemicals are used in dyes, bleaches, and straighteners, and small amounts may be absorbed through the skin. This has not been shown to affect the baby or cause miscarriage unless you are working with them every day in large quantities. For instance, cosmetologists have much more exposure to these chemicals, and may have a slightly greater risk of miscarriage than the average woman, according to some studies. However, this information as it pertains to pregnant salon employees is not conclusive because other factors besides the number of bleaches and permanents per week may be more important, such as standing more than eight hours a day and working more than forty hours per week.

Bad air quality, even the hazardous pollution after 9/11, has not been shown to increase miscarriages, at least not in the year after September 11, 2001. Mold, dust, and other airborne particles may cause disease and allergy as well, but are not associated with miscarriage.

## Food Poisoning

Different foodstuffs have been raised as a potential source for miscarriage because of certain chemicals contained within them. For instance, certain fish, like mackerel or tuna, raise concerns because they may contain high levels of mercury. Mercury in substantial amounts can cause miscarriage and fetal malformations. Also concerning are high levels of **PCBs** in farm-raised salmon. None of these have been associated with miscarriage directly, but there is a possible risk of malformation. Moderate use of these fish, as well as tilefish and shark, not more than three times a week while pregnant, is prudent.

## pcbs

Polychlorinated biphenyls (PCBs) are synthetic compounds that are the poisonous leftovers from toxic industrial chemicals, which were banned in the United States in 1977. However, PCBs still exist in many areas of the environment, and are commonly found in the bottom of rivers and lakes. They build up in the fatty tissue of certain fish and, although are not known to be generally harmful in small doses to the average person, they can cause birth defects and possibly miscarriage if consumed in large quantities.

Caffeine is another substance with a bad reputation in pregnancy, and this is mostly due to the fact that the information we have on caffeine is not definitive. In some research, more than two cups of coffee per day has been associated with an increase in miscarriages. Tea was not studied, but despite its seemingly milder reputation, it actually contains even more caffeine per cup than coffee (unless, of course, it is decaffeinated). It isn't likely that coffee drinking in moderation creates an increased risk for miscarriage, but you should avoid extreme amounts of caffeine in general. Most people will certainly drink fewer than three cups per day. Soft drinks, especially colas, are often consumed in large quantities but check the labels for caffeine in them, too, if you're drinking more than six servings a day. Just to show you how uncertain the information is, we're not even sure if the link is caffeine or coffee.

Food poisoning is always a concern during pregnancy, and it's understandable how some women can become extremely leery of whatever arrives in front of them on a plate. Restaurants are the most common sources of food poisoning. Food poisoning comes from bacterial products in contaminated foodstuffs. While it can certainly make you sick, risk of miscarriage occurs only in the most

severe cases, such as cholera, which you are not at all likely to contract unless you travel abroad to a place where it is prevalent. With
that said, though, pregnant women do need to be aware of toxic
agents in order to protect their babies and themselves. Any sign
of infection, especially fever, should be reported to your doctor.
Prompt diagnosis and treatment can make an enormous difference. Also, people with food allergies or on special diets, such as
gluten-free with celiac disease, can maintain their special requirements during pregnancy.

## WHAT CAN BE DONE

When it comes to the risk of toxic agents threatening pregnancy,
the good news is that there are many things that are within your
control, and others that you simply shouldn't lose any sleep over
because the risk is minuscule at best. Smoking, drinking, and illegal drugs are just not acceptable if you want to ensure the best possible outcome for your pregnancy—a healthy child and a healthy
mother. Prescribed and over-the-counter non-prescription medications should be discussed with your doctor, and only those approved should be taken. And of course, you can use the FDA
classification system outlined in this chapter as a guide. As for
herbal remedies and supplements, they should be avoided in pregnancy. They may seem harmless, and you may even swear up and
down the block that a certain supplement has relieved or improved
a particular malady, but the fact is, they have not been studied and
their risk as related to pregnancy is often unknown. They may be
harmful or they may not be—no one knows for sure. They may
combine with each other or with medications unpredictably, and
those effects can be severe, as in the serotonin syndrome or other
still-unrecognized illnesses.

Don't worry about X-rays and diagnostic imaging with magnetic resonance imaging or ultrasound—these are all safe. However,
even with that said, they should be kept to a minimum because the
effects are cumulative over your lifetime for X-rays. Chemical

exposure can be harmful to your own health and care should be taken to avoid excess exposure, but everyday chemicals are not associated with miscarriage, and the things that you use around the house are generally safe. And if you've been dyeing your hair all along, don't worry about continuing to do so. Hair treatments are not hazardous if you are getting them, and may slightly increase miscarriage risk only if you are giving them several times a day, 40 hours per week. If you do work in a salon, make sure the room you work in has proper ventilation, wear gloves, take frequent breaks in your work schedule, and when you need to eat, do so outside of your work area. These precautions should help reduce any risk of pregnancy loss from chemicals.

As for risk of food poisoning or consumption of toxic substances like PCBs, use common sense. Food should be refrigerated, cooked, and eaten only when it is properly washed and prepared. Eating out is a matter of knowing that the restaurant is acceptable to the health department of your community. If in doubt, do not eat out! Food poisoning is usually over in 24 to 48 hours. If at home you get nausea, vomiting, and diarrhea call your doctor, drink lots of fluids, and do not worry; it will not cause a miscarriage. If you are traveling in the Third World, food poisoning may well be dangerous. In this instance, see a doctor right away if you have symptoms. That environment could be very toxic.

When you're pregnant, the world outside your door (and, sometimes, even inside it!) can suddenly seem full of hazards to your baby. While there's nothing wrong with exercising caution—whether it be with food, chemicals, radiation exposure, or any other potentially hazardous substance or situation—just remember this: the baby is in the safe and protected environment inside you, and it takes quite a lot to put that environment at risk. Err on the side of caution in general, and always consult your doctor or midwife. Pregnancy loss is not likely as long as you follow my basic advice, and you and your baby should be just fine.

# twenty-three

## TRAUMA: DANGER ZONES

~~~~~~~~~~~~~~~~~~~~~~~~~~~~~~~~~~~~~~~~~~~~~~~~~

## MARYANNE

IT WAS ONE-THIRTY IN THE MORNING ON JANUARY 1, New Year's Day. Maryanne was driving home from a party, and her husband, Francis, was dozing next to her in spite of the salsa music she had blaring from the radio in order to stay awake. Francis had enjoyed the party, drinking and celebrating the new year feeling safe with the knowledge that Maryanne was the designated driver that night—after all, she was three months pregnant. The only alcohol that touched her lips was when she and Francis shared a midnight kiss.

She was concentrating on the road, driving home to Rockville Center, Long Island, as carefully as she could. An early rain had ended by that afternoon, but nightfall had turned the roads to black ice, making them as black and shiny as the top of the Lucite cocktail table at the party they just left, she thought. To be extra careful, Maryanne was taking the side streets home, avoiding the Sunrise Highway and the other returning revelers navigating their way on that slippery road.

There was no warning. The other car came through the intersection without stopping at the stop sign. It hit them someplace on the driver's side. When she came to, Maryanne was in the hospital. Francis, who had been bruised and cut, was standing at her bedside. He held her hand and explained what the doctors had told him: She had a concussion, a ruptured spleen, and a fractured pelvis. And they lost the baby.

## OVERCOMING THE PROBLEM

Maryanne told me this harrowing story when she came for a consultation about getting pregnant again. A year had passed and she had healed. She was missing her spleen and her pelvic bones looked slightly asymmetrical on an X-ray that she brought to me. She felt ready for another try at pregnancy—emotionally healed but worried about her risk of miscarriage after all that trauma. Would she be able to hold a pregnancy and deliver normally with all that injury and surgery, a blood transfusion, and a damaged but healed pelvis?

Other than her accident, Maryanne's medical history was normal. She had missed her period for five months after the accident because of her post-traumatic stress, but it had now returned to her normal cycle. Her physical examination was normal, except for the large scar on her abdomen where her spleen had been, a physical reminder of the accident. It wouldn't affect a future pregnancy, I advised her. I ordered blood tests to check on her hormonal status and the routine pre-pregnancy studies. They all were well within the normal range.

Sometimes, abdominal trauma or surgery will heal with scarring that blocks or restricts the normal motion of the **fallopian tubes**. That blockage can interfere with the oviduct's ability to sweep over the surface of the ovary and suck up the egg. The egg may not reach the tube and be fertilized. The egg can also become trapped in the tube by scarring and turn into an ectopic pregnancy. (See Chapter 11.)

---

### fallopian tubes

Also called oviducts, these are the flexible, moving structures that carry the released eggs, or ova, from the ovaries to the uterus.

---

I wanted to rule this out for Maryanne, so I also obtained a hysterosalpingogram, which is an X-ray procedure in which dye is injected through the vagina into the cervix and uterus and out the fallopian tubes. This outlined the uterus to rule out scar tissue as a possible problem and confirmed that the tubes were open. Her uterus was back to normal and her oviducts were not blocked by scar tissue. The abdominal injuries and the surgery that corrected them had healed very well.

I gave Maryanne and Francis the thumbs-up signal to try to get pregnant. Of course, things aren't always as easy as getting a green light. While her first pregnancy happened in a flash (within two months, she told me during our initial consultation), it was taking months to conceive a second time, even with no sign of blockage or scarring, and the rest of her tests coming back normal. They were both beginning to wonder if maybe some yet-unknown factor was affecting Maryanne's fertility after everything that happened that terrible New Year's night. One afternoon, she phoned me at my office asking if maybe she should have more tests to make sure she wasn't having other infertility issues. I advised her that only 50 percent of couples conceive in the first six months and that, although it was understandable that after such great physical trauma she'd be worried, there was no reason to worry just yet. I gave her three more months to try before a laparoscopy would be needed to look directly at her organs, and she uncomfortably agreed.

As it turned out, that laparoscopic surgery wasn't necessary at all. One month after that phone call, I got another from Maryanne: she was pregnant—and very pleased and relieved. After a normal pregnancy, she delivered at one week before her due date. Little Marybeth Francine was a healthy, 7½ lb girl and just perfect.

## WHAT CAN BE DONE?

Serious trauma in pregnancy like Maryanne's carries a high risk for both miscarriage and preterm birth. The most common causes are:

> motor vehicle accidents
> falling at home or outside the home
> physical abuse

Also, there is the rare occasion when severe trauma is inflicted by an animal, like a household pet. There are isolated tales of a dog or cat jumping on your abdomen and causing a miscarriage. There are no scientific reports to confirm those stories. Boating or swimming accidents are also rare, but still happen on occasion.

While pregnancy loss due to some kind of physical mishap is certainly an overused plot device on TV and in movies, it's believable for a reason. Trauma requiring a hospitalization is associated with complications of pregnancy and especially with miscarriage. The worst outcomes are those cases where the trauma is severe enough to lose the pregnancy during that hospitalization. But even with an all-clear from the hospital, a pregnant patient still holds a high risk of subsequent loss or preterm birth in the weeks after the traumatic event. That means that after discharge from the hospital the recovered patient is still in danger of miscarriage. She should be followed closely for bleeding, leakage of amniotic fluid, normal growth of the fetus, and normal appearance of the placenta on sonograms and signs of preterm labor.

As I mentioned earlier, vehicular accidents are the most common form of physical trauma for a pregnant woman. While you can't control everything that happens on the road, you can diligently adhere to a few well-known but vital safety precautions to up the ante on your baby's safety. Always remember to wear your seat belt. However, the seat belt should be placed across your hips and not across your abdomen when you are pregnant. Across the abdomen increases the risk of injury to the pregnant uterus and fetus.

And while this advice might seem obvious, it bears repeating: never get in a car with a driver who has been drinking. Of course, you shouldn't do this even if you are not pregnant; but as a pregnant woman, you aren't just risking your own life, but the pregnancy you are carrying, as well. To be considered legally impaired in the United States, your blood alcohol content (BAC) would be above .08 percent. Just to give you an idea of how alcohol impairs a person's ability, look at the following charts to see how quickly a drink or two or three can put someone past the legal limit:

## METABOLIC DRINKING RATES

### FOR MALES

| NUMBER OF DRINKS | BODY WEIGHT | | | | | | |
| --- | --- | --- | --- | --- | --- | --- | --- |
| | 100lbs | 125lbs | 150lbs | 175lbs | 200lbs | 225lbs | 250lbs |
| 1 | .043 | .034 | .029 | .025 | .022 | .019 | .017 |
| 2 | .087 | .069 | .058 | .050 | .043 | .039 | .035 |
| 3 | .130 | .103 | .087 | .075 | .065 | .058 | .052 |
| 4 | .174 | .139 | .116 | .100 | .087 | .078 | .070 |
| 5 | .217 | .173 | .145 | .125 | .108 | .097 | .087 |
| 6 | .261 | .209 | .174 | .150 | .130 | .117 | .105 |
| 7 | .304 | .242 | .203 | .175 | .152 | .136 | .122 |
| 8 | .348 | .278 | .232 | .200 | .174 | .156 | .139 |
| 9 | .391 | .312 | .261 | .225 | .195 | .175 | .156 |
| 10 | .435 | .346 | .290 | .250 | .217 | .198 | .173 |

## FOR FEMALES

| NUMBER OF DRINKS | BODY WEIGHT | | | | | | |
|---|---|---|---|---|---|---|---|
| | 100lbs | 125lbs | 150lbs | 175lbs | 200lbs | 225lbs | 250lbs |
| 1 | .050 | .040 | .034 | .029 | .026 | .022 | .020 |
| 2 | .101 | .080 | .068 | .058 | .050 | .045 | .041 |
| 3 | .152 | .120 | .101 | .087 | .078 | .068 | .061 |
| 4 | .203 | .162 | .135 | .117 | .101 | .091 | .082 |
| 5 | .253 | .202 | .169 | .146 | .126 | .113 | .010 |
| 6 | .234 | .244 | .203 | .175 | .152 | .136 | .122 |
| 7 | .355 | .282 | .237 | .204 | .177 | .159 | .142 |
| 8 | .406 | .324 | .271 | .233 | .203 | .182 | .162 |
| 9 | .456 | .364 | .304 | .262 | .227 | .207 | .182 |
| 10 | .507 | .404 | .338 | .292 | .253 | .227 | .202 |

## THE TIME FACTOR

| HOURS SINCE FIRST DRINK | SUBTRACT THIS FROM BAC |
|---|---|
| 1 | .015 |
| 2 | .030 |
| 3 | .045 |
| 4 | .060 |
| 5 | .075 |
| 6 | .090 |

From: *The Encyclopedia of Alcoholism* by Glen Evans and Robert O'Brien.
Copyright © 1991 by Facts on File, Inc., an imprint of Infobase Publishing. Reprinted with permission of the publisher.

Women are more susceptible to alcohol, just as your mom warned. Two drinks will do it for an average woman, so be careful if your best girlfriend drives you home, even if she has only been "lightly" drinking.

Whenever it's necessary, you should be the designated driver if your partner or companion for an evening out has consumed too much. And if you don't or can't drive the car for some reason, ask your host for the number of a reliable cab service. The extra fee is well worth your life.

Another important thing to keep in mind for every pregnant woman is that your body is different and your balance is thrown off by the time you are halfway through pregnancy. Your usual activities, exercise routines, and travel are all affected by the change in your body configuration. This change produces a new center of gravity, as well as a new shape of your body. You will bump into things, and you are more likely to have an unexpected fall—in fact, 25 percent of trauma during pregnancy is due to a fall of some sort. Even getting in and out of the bathtub or stepping off the curb may cause you to fall because of this shift in the normal center of gravity of your body. Simply put, you must be more cautious and aware of your surroundings when you are pregnant. There is a world of experience that tells us that a pregnant woman must be more careful during her daily routine (and that people should help a pregnant woman with her activities!). It isn't called a delicate condition for nothing.

The most disturbing cause of trauma and subsequent pregnancy loss in America is one that is inflicted on a pregnant woman due to abuse and domestic violence. This is a totally preventable cause of pregnancy loss. No woman should tolerate an abusive relationship; least of all should she tolerate it when she is pregnant. Get help and get out if you are one of these women. There are hotlines to agencies for battered women in every city and emergency police numbers to call. The following are a few helpful resources:

- National Mental Health Information Center,
  http://www.mentalhealth.samhsa.gov
- National Coalition Against Domestic Violence,
  http://www.ncadv.org
- Domestic Violence & Mental Health Policy Initiative,
  http://www.dvmhpi.org

- CDC's National Center for Injury Prevention and Control, http://www.cdc.gov/ncipc
- Black Women's Health Imperative, http://www.blackwomenshealth.org
- The National Center for Victims of Crime, http://www.ncvc.org
- Rape, Abuse, and Incest National Network (RAINN), http://www.rainn.org
- Witness Justice, http://www.witnessjustice.org

At the very least, there is one number that is the same in every city—911.

The best news, however, is that only 27 percent of pregnancies complicated by severe maternal injuries will result in miscarriage—that's just slightly worse than the number of pregnancies ending in miscarriage in general. Even with severe trauma to a pregnant woman, such as broken bones or injury requiring surgery, nearly three-quarters of women will not lose their baby. As for minor injuries, such as a fall with bruising, or even whiplash from a motor vehicle accident, these add only a small increase to the risk of miscarriage. It's so small, in fact, as to be insignificant when we try to measure it in studies, so a bump or a minor injury will not cause miscarriage. The best advice to follow when you are pregnant is to err on the side of caution: always wear your seat belt placed across your hips and not across your pregnant tummy; be careful not only when you are out and about, but even when at home doing your normal things (especially in and out of the bathtub).

If you have experienced severe trauma from an accident in the past, do what Maryanne did—have a thorough dialogue with your physician and make sure you have the green light to go forward with another pregnancy. That is the best way to make sure that you and your baby will be healthy. Remember the odds are way on your side.

# twenty-four

## STRESS, PSYCHOLOGY, AND PREGNANCY

~~~~~~~~~~~~~~~~~~~~~~~~~~~~~~~~~~~~~~~~~~~~~~~~~

## MADELINE

MADELINE WALKED INTO MY CONSULTING ROOM VISIBLY
annoyed. She had waited five minutes past her scheduled appointment and showed the impatience of someone accustomed to getting things done with no delay. Greeting her, I apologized for the
delay and asked how I might help. She icily replied, "I don't know
that you can help me."

I asked her to tell me about her problems to see if I could at
least answer her questions. She accepted that grudgingly. When
she began to tell me about what had brought her to my office that
afternoon, I could understand why she was so angry. Our discussion revealed that Madeline had lost a baby at 40 weeks, a full-
term baby. There had been no explanation given to her. Two years
ago, Madeline was 36 years old and pregnant for the first time. She
was one day past her due date when she realized that she had felt
no fetal movement all day. She became alarmed and called her doctor, who told her to go to the hospital. There was no fetal heartbeat
when she got there. Labor was induced that night, and 24 hours
later there was the stillbirth of a normal baby girl. "She looked like
she was sleeping," Madeline said, her voice catching in a near sob.
They found nothing, not even a cord around the neck of the baby.
It was just an unanswered question. Madeline was left with grief
and a guilty feeling when they said that it was from stress.

Madeline was the executive editor at one of the top magazines in New York and supervised a large, ambitious staff. It was a high-powered job, but she tolerated it well. You might even say she thrived on the excitement that came along with deadlines, constant meetings, trips abroad, and tight schedules. She was generally healthy and had an uneventful pregnancy until the baby died. Her family history revealed only heart disease in her father, but otherwise nothing relevant. Madeline's husband, Donald, was also an ambitious, type-A personality, just like his wife: he worked for an investment bank and traveled worldwide. As for his health, he had ulcerative colitis and was constantly under medical care, and colitis and colon cancer ran in his family. That was not related, either, except that it seemed likely that she was not getting much emotional support from her husband given his own medical problems; maybe she did not need it.

I asked her if she might be thinking about another pregnancy, and she said, "Maybe, after I hear what you have to say, or maybe not." Madeline was not a woman who allowed shades of gray into her life, so I took this to mean that she wanted me to evaluate her chances for a healthy baby if she again conceived. I advised her that we needed a full diagnostic workup in order to get her the answers she needed. She agreed, and her physical examination was totally normal. Great news, of course, but slightly disappointing to Madeline because it didn't lead to any clues about why she suffered such a terrible pregnancy loss. I sent for her previous records and any tests done on the fetus. Then I ordered blood tests to be done, looking for possible causes of stillbirth. I was searching for an answer—for hormonal problems, auto-immune diseases, infections, blood diseases, clotting defects, antiphospholipid syndrome, and even syphilis (although I did not mention that one to her); I hoped that the answer had to be out there somewhere.

## OVERCOMING THE PROBLEM

All of the fetal tests from two years ago were negative, I told Madeline at the next visit. The records were not revealing. The fetus had not been autopsied, nor were there samples taken from it for study. There had been no cord around the neck, no separation of the placenta, and no cultures for viruses or bacteria taken. The tests that I had done for her had just one hint of a possibility. The **antinuclear antibody** (**ANA**) was weakly positive. This was the only clue to the mystery of a stillbirth said to be caused by stress.

---

## antinuclear antibody (ana)

The ANA is a blood test that is often positive in patients with auto-immune diseases and the level rises as the disease gets worse.

---

I repeated the ANA and ordered more tests looking for evidence of an active auto-immune disease that might have caused the death of Madeline's baby, such as systemic lupus erythematosus, rheumatoid arthritis, or dermatomyositis. The blood tests for **complement,** rheumatoid factor, high sedimentation rate, antiphospholipid antibodies, and elevated immunoglobulins were within the normal range, but the ANA remained positive at a dilution of 1:40. The test stayed positive even when the blood was diluted with water 40 times the size of the sample. That level is not diagnostic and sometimes is present when there is no disease at all.

---

## complement

Part of the immune system, which is often abnormal in the blood of patients with auto-immune disease, especially with systemic lupus.

---

I asked Madeline to see one of my colleagues who specialized in auto-immune diseases and to come back with her husband for a discussion after that. The report from our consultant confirmed my findings. No apparent disease, just a positive test.

She and Donald arrived together a week later. He was dressed in typical power-broker fashion: a charcoal-gray suit and a blue shirt with a white collar, yellow and navy striped tie, and an intense look that went well with prematurely graying hair. I explained that although Madeline and Donald both lived in a high-powered and high-stress environment, it was not likely that stress caused the pregnancy loss. A look of relief came over him as he heard my words, and his face visibly softened as he relaxed in his chair.

Madeline was also dressed perfectly for her role as a high-powered magazine executive, but she was not as quick to wear the same look of relief as her husband. Her brown eyes narrowed as she leaned toward me in her chair: "How can I be sure it won't happen again?" she asked through tight lips, her teeth nearly clenched. I looked into her anxious face and told Madeline that I would do everything in my power as a physician to prevent it. I told the couple that there would be lots of stress along the way in her next pregnancy, no matter what I did, but stress—no matter how much of it she was under—would *not* cause her to miscarry; nor had it caused her to lose her first pregnancy. I told her that until she had safely given birth to a healthy newborn, stress would be a factor, especially coming off the terrible loss she had already suffered, but together we could handle it.

Madeline took a long, deep breath, and closed her eyes as she exhaled. When she opened them again, they had softened and were shiny, almost with tears. The tight lines around her mouth vanished as she finally said: "I believe you." Six months later, she was pregnant again.

Her blood tests were normal, except for the ANA, which remained at 1:40, the same borderline-positive result, but clearly persistent and not just a non-specific finding. Her sonogram showed an eight-week fetus with a strong heartbeat. Madeline was both unbelieving that she was pregnant and fearful that she would miscarry. Her contradictory feelings gave her more stress than usual, and I certainly couldn't blame her. It showed in her posture and her tight-lipped smile, a forced sort of grin, when I told her that it all was looking just fine. "Will it stay fine?" she asked. I did my best to reassure her and try to keep Madeline in a positive state of mind. "So far, so good," I replied. "We are off to a good start."

I outlined our plan for her: close follow-up on her pregnancy with visits and monthly sonograms, blood tests every two months, a fetal echocardiogram to evaluate the fetal heart function at 20, 28, and 32 weeks of pregnancy, fetal kick counts daily after 28 weeks, weekly fetal well-being studies beginning 8 weeks before the due date, and finally, a scheduled delivery about two weeks early, or sooner, if a problem arose. In other words, Madeline and her baby were under intensive surveillance for any problems, and careful evaluation of the mom for the appearance of any disease process that could affect the outcome. Accustomed to dealing with schedules and long-term, well-thought-out plans, this suited Madeline just fine. She had me repeat the plan and entered all the information into her BlackBerry, a device she was never without.

The pregnancy progressed very well. The baby's growth and activity were normal for the beginning and middle of pregnancy in spite of Madeline's unrelenting stress and worry. She kept working at her usual torrid pace at the magazine because, she told me, it distracted her from her bad thoughts about losing another baby. My suspicions about Donald's abilities as a supportive partner were correct and he acted in what I came to know as his usual unsupportive self. In fact, his colitis acted up from the stress on him. Madeline had to support him while he refused hospitalization but consented to stay home and take off two weeks from his high-tension job. Talk about stress during your pregnancy!

The only abnormalities were a persistent blood level of 1:40 for Madeline's ANA and, toward the last part of pregnancy, a fetus just below average size for the dates of measurement, but still growing. At 38 weeks, I initiated a scheduled induction of labor. Thankfully,

Donald realized his wife really needed his support and he was there for the birth, having made arrangements not to travel to the London office that week. He did not seem to be at all worried and was very eager for the process to start. I'd even say he was excited.

Madeline, on the other hand, was frightened and very tense. She suffered a very hard labor, even with her epidural, and after pushing for two hours in the second stage of labor was exhausted. After 16 hours of labor, I delivered with forceps a very healthy little girl. Lauren Elizabeth was 5 lb 15 oz, and two weeks early—but her parents didn't seem to mind. The ordeal was over at last.

At the four-week follow-up visit, I repeated the ANA test, and it was higher at 1:80, but still there were no symptoms of any disease. My guess was that Madeline had an underlying tendency to develop an auto-immune disease in the future, and I advised her to be checked regularly by her general doctor, especially for joint pains, rashes, or any kidney or lung problems.

The following year, her internist called to tell me that she had diagnosed Madeline with **systemic lupus erythematosus,** an auto-immune disease. When Madeline came to see me next, she was taking prednisone, a steroid drug for the treatment of her systemic lupus. She was seeing me because she wanted to talk about her next pregnancy.

---

### systemic lupus erythematosus
A generalized auto-immune disease that damages joints, skin, lungs, kidneys, and other organs.

---

## CAN STRESS AFFECT PREGNANCY?
An unexplained fetal death is one of the most devastating experiences anyone might have. Unfortunately, it is often unexplained because the search for the explanation is incomplete, as in

Madeline's case. When the investigation is unrevealing, the patient is often told that the cause must have been stress.

Let us get this fact clear right here and now: *stress alone has never been shown to cause fetal loss,* whether the case be miscarriage or fetal death. There has been evidence for preterm birth and smaller-than-average birth weight, but there are usually many other factors along with stress that can be related to these outcomes. Babies are born to women in concentration camps, during periods of war, poverty, and famine, and to women in prisons, without evidence for stress alone as a cause for miscarriage. One study of 23 women who had repeated miscarriages found high levels of the stress hormones cortisone and urocortin, not in the mother's blood, but in the lost fetus's and in the uterus. But this suggests local stress hormones in the fetus due to its stress from the process of miscarriage. If the stress caused the miscarriage, the mother's blood should show the high levels of stress hormones, and it did not.

Psychosocial studies have found more stressful events in the two weeks before a miscarriage than in women who did not miscarry, but this is subject to recall errors, emphasizing the bad memories of a recent miscarriage compared with a normal birth nine months later. Studies showing high levels of cortisol, a stress hormone, in the urine of women who miscarried in the first trimester, cannot distinguish between cause and effect. The high cortisol is as likely to be due to having symptoms of a miscarriage as to being the cause of the miscarriage. What this means for you and what is most important to take away from this chapter is this: there is still no proof that stress causes miscarriage.

Madeline's case is a very good example. She had high stress levels in her first pregnancy due to her work, her husband's equally stressful work, and his refusal to deal with his chronic illness. Imagine what the stress level must have been like in her second pregnancy, after the horrible experience with her first. In the second pregnancy, she had her only previous pregnancy experience ending in a fetal death. The cause was still unclear, but she repeatedly had been told that it was stress and she should relax—which, of course, only serves to make a person feel even more stressed. Her job was the same, since she did not stop working, and her husband was sicker than before, maybe due to the stress on him. Colitis, Donald's disease, often acts up with stress. He was not only unsupportive; Madeline had to help him since he refused hospitalization. Then, in this second pregnancy, there were constant tests and induced hard labor. How about that for stress?

Still, Madeline had a normal, healthy baby with more stress than she had in the first pregnancy. One year later, we found the reason. It was systemic lupus erythematosus first showing itself as a fetal loss, a well-known problem with that disease. There was a cause, after all—and it was not stress.

## WHAT CAN BE DONE

The approach to a problem like Madeline's is to look for the cause. Late miscarriage or fetal death can be caused by serious infections with a virus, such as cytomegalovirus or bacteria like brucellosis, among others. These and other infections are discussed in Chapter 21. Blood tests can look for these, as well as testing the fetus and taking cultures from it. Samples taken from the stillborn, or an autopsy, if possible, can reveal the cause. Samples of blood and tissue for genetic, viral, and bacterial studies often provide an answer to unexplained stillbirths when they are taken from the stillborn fetus.

In addition, maternal blood tests should be done for thrombophilias and maternal diseases, such as **platelet antibodies** or auto-immune diseases, such as the systemic lupus that was found in Madeline's case. Maternal vaginal cultures and blood tests should be done for possible infectious causes at the time of any late pregnancy loss, and the parents' blood type should be checked to look for incompatibilities, including platelet antibodies and rare antibodies, such as anti-P, which is associated with miscarriage. With a correct diagnosis, appropriate treatment is begun before pregnancy. Even so, no diagnosis may be clear, or it could be borderline as in Madeline's initial case. What then for anxious parents-to-be?

## platelet antibodies

The pregnant woman makes antibodies against the fetus blood platelets. This occurs when the platelets contain a factor contributed by the father that is absent in the mother's blood. The result is destruction of the fetal blood platelets, which causes fetal bleeding and death of the fetus in the uterus or in labor.

It is important not only to perform appropriate diagnostic tests post–pregnancy loss, but to repeat them. As with Madeline, the diagnostic evaluation is done before the next pregnancy and repeated in early pregnancy. Blood tests for hormonal problems, antibody and auto-immune issues, thrombophilia, and infectious diseases are done again in the first trimester. Cultures are obtained from the mother's vagina and evaluated for infectious agents. Close follow-up is needed, with frequent sonograms every month to make sure that fetal growth is progressing normally and a fetal echocardiogram to assess the fetal heart function. Once the mother can feel fetal movements, fetal kick counts can be done for the same one-hour period every night. If there are no fetal movements for that hour, the patient waits for a second hour and counts during that time. If there are still no fetal movements, she is seen for a sonogram and a **nonstress test** immediately. When the fetal movements occur at least three times in that hour, the patient is reassured that her baby is well.

> ## nonstress test
> A fetal heart rate test to evaluate fetal well-being by observing increases in the fetal heart rate associated with fetal movements.

Later on, weekly biophysical profile tests using ultrasound to measure amniotic fluid and fetal movements are done starting at 34 weeks of pregnancy, and umbilical artery Doppler studies are done to evaluate blood flow between the fetus and the placenta. Finally, when the fetus is mature enough, or when amniocentesis shows satisfactory lung development, delivery is planned. With careful management, women who experienced a previous stillbirth almost never have another tragedy like that.

Medical evidence supports the concept that a stillbirth usually has a medical reason, such as the trauma of a car accident or an underlying disease, and that often the cause will appear years later. If it is looked for, the cause can often be found and corrected. I do not believe that stress alone can cause a pregnancy loss.

Since the tragic events of our recent history, pregnant women in America have been coping with stress more and more. Military women returning from Vietnam and Iraq with post-traumatic stress disorder, and civilians in New York City after the horror of September 11, 2001, did not experience a higher miscarriage rate than usual. Still, everyone needs to cope with stress in life. How do we know when we are stressed? We feel drained and exhausted, lack appetite, energy, and sexual interest, and do not sleep well. Of course, these symptoms are common during a normal pregnancy. Pregnant women are normally anxious about themselves and their baby. With the addition of stress, though, the symptoms get worse. You may feel numb, sad, irritable, and unable to concentrate. What to do about it?

Ask to be comforted. Ask your spouse, family, friends, clergy, and doctor. Talk about your feelings and worries. Try stress-reduction techniques like slow breathing and muscle relaxation exercises, meditation, or just take some time—if only a few minutes every day—to calm your mind and relax comfortably in a quiet place. If necessary, a psychologist or psychiatrist can help. Remember that talking it out *is* therapy. Stress is part of life and is increased when you are pregnant, but it has little to do with miscarriage.

# section five

UNDERSTANDING

# twenty-five

## GRIEVING, COPING, HOPING

~~~~~~~~~~~~~~~~~~~~~~~~~~~~~~~~~~~~~~~~

MISCARRIAGE AT ANY STAGE OF PREGNANCY CREATES A deep feeling of loss. The grief, guilt, loss of self-confidence, and depression are universal. Some individuals may experience acute stress disorders, as well. One study shows a 7 percent incidence of typical post-traumatic stress disorder at four months after a miscarriage. Psychologists and psychiatrists agree that the most devastating loss of all, more than loss of a parent, a spouse, or a sister or brother, is the loss of a child. To a pregnant woman and to some husbands, as well, although their child was not born, the trauma is the same.

Most couples fantasize about the fetus and it becomes more real as pregnancy progresses. For the mother-to-be, this is even more intense as she experiences the physical changes to her body. You feel yourself change. Add to that the knowledge that you and your partner have created something that, no matter how small, is growing in your womb—it's clearly a very intense experience for a woman.

Contemporary obstetrics introduces the fetus at five or six weeks of pregnancy through the visual aid of an ultrasound machine, and a bond is formed. By eight or ten weeks, a tiny person is seen, enhanced by the eagerness of the parents, the enthusiasm of the sonographer, and the power of the human imagination. I often joke with an expectant couple about the small creature on the screen, only nine or ten weeks old. "I think it looks like Dad," I sometimes say, even though it is only two inches long. Because it has become so real so early in pregnancy, a miscarriage is perceived by most couples as the death of a child. When there is repeated loss, the couple adds self-doubt, anger, and a need to blame to the cauldron of emotion already boiling within them. It must be someone's fault, they rationalize.

Although some people may feel numb at first after a miscarriage, it is very normal to experience grief. These intense feelings have to be let out somehow and not held back. The psychological stress must be expressed to be relieved. Pregnancy is not only a major physical event in a woman's life, but a major psychological one, as well. It is a milestone. When a woman anticipates motherhood, it invests her with self-actualization and she gains the power that she has always believed her own mother held—the proverbial passing of the torch. Every culture acknowledges the awe-inspiring creative power embodied in a mother. In West Africa, the Yoruba tribe has an annual celebration of nationhood, based on four sources of power. These are represented by four giant Epa masks, worn on the shoulders of the ceremony dancers. They are masks of the King, the Warrior, the Farmer, and the Mother. Equal to the other three, the Mother is recognized as one of the four great powers of the Yoruba nation.

## GRIEVING

In spite of the reasonable observation that "it's not your fault," when the anticipated motherhood and all that it symbolizes has vanished, its power unrealized, it leaves the woman with immense feelings of failure. Add to that the profound sadness and feelings of inadequacy and deprivation that follow, and the result is the grieving process. All these feelings are magnified and an anxiety state is added when the miscarriages recur.

The grieving process has been intensively studied by psychiatrists and psychologists. In general, there are three phases:

1. Denial phase
2. Mourning phase
3. Recovery phase

Both expectant parents may go through this process, but the father generally is less affected because the psychology of motherhood is far more complex and intense than that of fatherhood. However, when the miscarriage occurs after the first three months of pregnancy, the man's involvement with the pregnancy and his own ideas of fatherhood are greater, and it is not uncommon for him to have a strong grief reaction, as well.

Grieving varies with the stage of pregnancy when miscarriage occurs and with every individual. The presence of a formed fetus in a second- or third-trimester loss may actually be helpful in completing the process. Horrific as it sounds, in this instance we can use our rituals of death and its finality to allow a necessary cathartic close on a difficult and extremely painful experience. Loss of the perceived fetus during first-trimester miscarriage can be tricky, however. One can't participate in the appropriate rituals or tangibly mourn the imagined child. Many women feel adrift in this situation, without the anchor of typical mourning to hold her in place. Add to that the notion that friends and family, while sympathetic, may not recognize the amount of time a woman might need to mourn her loss, and thus not understand her grief or feelings of melancholy. Sometimes her husband or family or friends worry that talking about miscarriage or pregnancy will increase her grief, so they avoid the subject, and the woman winds up feeling utterly without support.

In whatever trimester the loss occurs, the three phases of grieving usually take place, each lasting a variable interval. For most women, the process takes about two or three months, but up to a year is not uncommon. The denial phase begins with a feeling of numbness and disbelief, and sometimes requires repeated sonograms and blood tests to convince the patient that her pregnancy is no more.

The mourning phase follows once the miscarriage is acknowledged, with feelings of sadness, failure, loss of self-esteem, and sometimes intense anger, hostility, and a need to place blame. The patient often looks for an explanation for the loss and frequently wonders about fault, most often in her own behavior. Guilt is expressed for excessive work, or for not eating properly, or for a past behavior like a voluntary pregnancy termination. The miscarriage is sometimes viewed as retribution for some imagined transgression. "Why did this happen to me?" is the most frequent question I hear and the most revealing. The patient often desperately needs an explanation and fears that it is somehow her fault.

All too often, another unfortunate factor is added to the mix, as well, in the form of the couple not discussing the pregnancy loss at all for fear of upsetting the other. They will avoid the subject because of the disturbing feeling that each may be blaming the other. This phase requires more support to encourage the expression of the emotions troubling the woman and very often troubling her husband, too.

Sadness, jealousy of other women with children, feelings of inadequacy and anger are gradually expressed and dealt with as the mourning phase enables the woman to accept her loss and begin to recover. During the mourning phase, patients have difficulty sleeping, feel fatigued, have less appetite, less libido, and may be irritable and depressed. As they enter the recovery phase, these symptoms will begin to fade away. Interest in life gradually returns, as they work out their loss and come to accept it. The recovery phase takes months to years, and for some people there is always a sadness tucked away somewhere in a corner of the heart.

## COPING

For a few couples, the mourning is permanent and may even be strong enough to end a marriage. When one partner becomes chronically depressed, when they blame each other, or do not communicate, the result is persistent pain for both. Sometimes the man will immediately try to offer solutions—a plan of action, a method to fix what is broken, attempted answers to unanswered questions—instead of just listening and relating to the feelings his partner has expressed. When the man is silent or tries to rationalize, it too often is interpreted by the woman to mean that he does not care. Of course, nothing could be further from the truth—in both of these instances, he just is not able to express his feelings because he has been trained to repress them. Men are conditioned to repress feelings in Western society and in many other cultures. Men are taught to be unemotional because that is seen as being strong. For both partners, stifling your feelings and avoiding the subject leaves the pain and bitterness of pregnancy loss unresolved, and may stifle the marriage in the end. You have to talk with each other. Sharing the pain and grieving together will strengthen the relationship and speed the recovery. Even for those couples who have suffered the misery of repeated losses, it is the shared bereavement that allows for healing the heart wounds of miscarriage.

In addition to each other, there are other sources of support to assist in recovery from the trauma of losing a baby. Your doctor and the nursing staff at the hospital should appreciate your emotional turmoil and be supportive from the outset. They may even offer counseling services at the hospital. Your religious faith and contact with your clergy can help, as well, and for many people their faith is an all-encompassing source of strength and comfort in a painful situation such as pregnancy loss. The Internet is a far-reaching source not only of articles and information, but also of message boards on Web sites like iVillage.com where women who have experienced miscarriage form virtual support groups. Family and friends should be comforting and not unwilling to discuss the miscarriage for fear of upsetting you, but you have to let them know that it is okay to talk about it. And if there are certain things you don't want to hear, and others you do, let them know. For instance, many women who experience pregnancy loss, especially multiple pregnancy loss, feel incredibly frustrated when loved ones offer suggestions like adoption, just relaxing, or any other "solution" to the problem. Be clear about your feelings: explain that what you need is someone to be supportive; that, of course, you've considered all the angles and are considering how to proceed, but really what you need is simply someone to listen. In fact, you need to talk about it when you are ready to get back to a normal life.

Sometimes, clinical depression will follow a pregnancy loss, especially if there have been others preceding it. A psychiatrist or a psychologist can help. Depression is an illness and there is very effective treatment. When your grief is prolonged, and you are not getting any better, you need to think about depression. The symptoms are the same, but more so: less energy, fatigue, absent libido, difficulty getting out of bed in the morning, sadness, feelings of worthlessness, loss of appetite, loss of weight, unwillingness to speak with friends and family, alcohol or other substance abuse, and inability to think about anything, including what you will do tomorrow. These symptoms mean that you need to see a mental-health professional. There is nothing shameful about needing medical help for a mental illness. It is a sickness, not a weakness, and it can be treated and even cured.

## HOPING

It is vital for you to believe and accept that after a miscarriage, grieving is normal. Trying to suppress it will not help you get back to your normal life, or back on track to becoming a parent. There is a process of recognizing the loss, feeling sad, guilty, and upset, and then returning to your normal life. That process is experienced by just about every couple following a lost pregnancy. Men and women cope with it differently, and the coping varies with different individuals and circumstances. A healthy woman will recover physically very rapidly, but emotional recovery takes time: months or even years. Everyone wants an explanation for how it happened, why it happened to them, and if it will happen again. Careful investigation of the miscarriage and complete evaluation of the couple will go a long way toward answering those questions. More than that, it often shows the way to preventing another miscarriage. Your doctor will do more than give you emotional support, because an accurate diagnosis will give you a realistic estimate of successful pregnancy next time and a means to get there.

Your emotional distress will have to be cleared up before you are willing to try again, and that varies with every person and every miscarriage. Ask to be comforted. Ask your spouse, your family, and your friends. Do not hesitate to talk about it for fear of stirring up the sadness, for yourself or your husband, or causing awkwardness for your loved ones. Talking about it and expressing your feelings soothes the pain. If the miscarriage was a terrible experience, filled with bleeding, pain, and emergency surgery in the middle of the night by a stranger in a strange and frightening place, you are at risk for post-traumatic stress. You will need to talk about it very badly, and a psychiatrist or psychologist will help you enormously. There are vast resources to help you to conquer the fear and anxiety over trying again. Even just once more, as you may promise yourself, may seem like more than you are ready for right now. That is okay; you need time and support to return to your normal self.

After a miscarriage, most couples find that their marriage is stronger, tempered by tragedy, as iron is strengthened by fire into steel. In a loving relationship, with a couple that shares their feelings and communicates with each other, the bond between them grows.

And so there is HOPE. After the pain, after the grieving, you *will* recover. And yes, you can be brave enough to try again. You will be healthy. You will be forearmed with knowledge of your problem and its proper treatment. You will have enormous support and a loving spouse beside you. You will banish self-doubt and be confident. And you will have your child.

# twenty-six

## FAQ: YOUR QUESTIONS ANSWERED

~~~~~~~~~~~~~~~~~~~~~~~~~~~~~~~~~~~~~~~~~~~~~~

SOMETIMES YOU JUST NEED TO KNOW THE ANSWER TO one question, one that burns on your mind, but for which you do not want a detailed discussion of the biology and the chemistry of the entire issue. This chapter tries to give you the quick answers to the most frequently asked questions. The subjects are covered in detail throughout this book, so more information is available to you if you want to cover the subject in depth. I have divided the questions into specific categories for easy access:

- Medical History
- Lifestyle
- Medical Interventions

So, if the question is about your medical history, including your family history, look under that heading. If it is about medical issues such as questions about amniocentesis or birth, check out Medical Interventions first, and if it is about your work or your activities, you should be able to find it under Lifestyle.

## MEDICAL HISTORY QUESTIONS

### Inherited Tendency to Miscarry
1. QUESTION: My mother had miscarriages before she had me. Can a tendency to miscarriage be inherited?

ANSWER: Yes, there are many studies that show miscarriages running in families, but there are numerous correctable causes that are familial. Presently, there are so many different causes that your mother's miscarriages will not predict your risk of miscarriage. As we learn more about human genetics, we will be able to pinpoint these abnormal genes and figure out what to do about them even better than our treatments today permit.

### Blood Clots

2. QUESTION: My family has problems with blood clots, and I was told that causes miscarriages. Can I have that problem?

ANSWER: There are specific inherited blood-clotting problems called thrombophilias. The only one specifically known to cause miscarriage is factor V Leiden mutation. Some others have been associated with miscarriage in some medical reports, but the information is not conclusive. You should ask your doctor to test you for these increased clotting disorders because you may need to avoid birth control pills when you are not pregnant and be on an anticoagulant of some sort when you are pregnant.

### Age Effects

3. QUESTION: Can my age cause miscarriages?

ANSWER: Age by itself is not a cause, but the risk of miscarriage increases over the age of 35 because there is a decrease in the number and quality of the eggs left in your ovaries. By age 40, most women have very few healthy eggs left, so miscarriages are more common, about one in three pregnancies, and only about ten percent of women in the 45 and older age group remain fertile.

### Man's Age

4. QUESTION: My husband is older. Can the man's age cause miscarriage?

ANSWER: The man's age has an effect on the miscarriage rate after the age of 40. For men over 40, the risk of a miscarriage is increased. It is thought to be due to a decrease in the sperm quality with aging.

### Semen Quality

5. QUESTION: My husband's semen analysis shows poor quality and motility (e.g., ability to move quickly). Does this cause miscarriage?

ANSWER: Sperm count, morphology, and motility are key factors in fertility. When the count is good, the morphology, which is how normal the sperm appear, and motility, which is how well they swim, become more important. A large number of abnormal sperm is believed to increase the risk of miscarriage. But when all factors are low, inability to conceive is the more common problem.

### Diabetes

6. QUESTION: I have diabetes, and my doctor says I am likely to miscarry. Is that true?

ANSWER: Diabetics have a greater risk of pregnancy loss, but you do not have to miscarry. When the diabetes is well controlled, your risk is about the same as the average woman without diabetes.

### Hypertension in Parents

7. QUESTION: Both my parents have high blood pressure. Do I have a higher risk of miscarriage?

ANSWER: You first need to know why they have high blood pressure. If they have a hereditary disease, you may get it, too. If you have high blood pressure, you are not more likely to miscarry, but you are more likely to deliver your baby early. You should check with your doctor and your parents to determine what the cause is for their high blood pressure, if it is a condition that is hereditary, and if you have it.

### Anemia

8. QUESTION: I have anemia and I am taking iron pills to build up my red blood cell count. Am I more likely to miscarry?

ANSWER: There are different kinds of anemia. If you have iron-deficiency anemia, you can cure it with iron, vitamin C, and folic acid before you get pregnant. Even if it persists in pregnancy, you are not more likely to miscarry, but there are other anemias that do increase pregnancy loss, such as sickle cell and thalassemia. You should see your doctor to be sure about the diagnosis, the right treatment, and the risks.

## Asthma

9. QUESTION: I have asthma and take medicine and use an inhaler. Can that cause a miscarriage?

ANSWER: Asthma and the different treatments do not cause miscarriage, but untreated asthma can be serious in pregnancy and can lead to preterm births. Be sure that your doctor has controlled your asthma before you get pregnant.

## Thyroid Disease

10. QUESTION: Every one of my sisters and myself have thyroid problems. One of them had a miscarriage, and I am worried about having one, too.

ANSWER: Both overactive and underactive thyroid glands can lead to a miscarriage. You need to see your doctor to get your thyroid in the proper state and on the right dosage of medication. Then, when you are pregnant, your thyroid function should be checked regularly. That will prevent miscarriage and avoid problems with the baby, as well.

## Bleeding

11. QUESTION: Does bleeding in pregnancy cause a miscarriage?

ANSWER: Bleeding in the first three months is associated with miscarriage in about half of the patients, but the other half do just fine. Bleeding later on can cause pregnancy loss as well, but only in about 2 to 5 percent of pregnancies is there later bleeding and a subsequent miscarriage.

## Abortion

**12. QUESTION:** Will having had a previous pregnancy termination cause a miscarriage when you want to have a baby?

**ANSWER:** One or two previous abortions, done in the first three months, will not increase the risk for a subsequent pregnancy. Three or more, or an abortion after fourteen weeks, has been associated with increased risk of miscarriage.

## Urinary Tract Infections

**13. QUESTION:** I keep getting urinary tract infections. If I get one while I am pregnant, can it make me miscarry?

**ANSWER:** In general, an ordinary kind of urinary tract infection will not cause a miscarriage. However, a very high fever or a kidney infection might do it; so prompt diagnosis and treatment are needed; otherwise, a simple bladder infection could find its way into your kidneys if untreated and produce a serious kidney infection.

## Vaginal Discharge

**14. QUESTION:** Since I got pregnant, I have a lot of whitish discharge. Does that mean that I could miscarry?

**ANSWER:** Increased discharge is common in pregnancy and is not a sign of miscarriage. Later on, a watery discharge or mucus may be a sign of early changing of the cervix. When it occurs in the second trimester or last three months, you should see your doctor to be sure that the baby is not born too early. Vaginitis and bacterial vaginosis do not cause miscarriage. They are common in pregnancy, as well as when you are not pregnant. They can cause annoying symptoms, and they can be treated while you are pregnant without fear of miscarriage. Sometimes, they may be associated with preterm birth, and that is why if you are having a discharge and it is persistent, it is wise to see your doctor or midwife and have a diagnosis made.

## Cramps

15. QUESTION: I keep having cramps since I got pregnant. Am I threatening to miscarry?

ANSWER: While cramps are common in early pregnancy, they do not usually mean miscarriage because they are mild contractions of your uterus. The uterus contracts throughout pregnancy on and off, irregularly. Cramps often disappear for days at a time in early pregnancy. The contractions get stronger and more frequent in the last two months of pregnancy, until they become effective, and that is how you go into labor. But, in early pregnancy, they are usually mild. If they are continuous over hours, getting stronger and more frequent, and especially if they are followed by bleeding, call your doctor because that may be a threatened miscarriage.

## Vomiting

16. QUESTION: I keep throwing up since I found out that I was pregnant. Will this make me lose the pregnancy?

ANSWER: Nausea and vomiting are frequent in the first three months and do not mean that miscarriage is likely. Rarely, they can be severe, and even then miscarriages are not increased. Very rarely, they are very severe and associated with an abnormal pregnancy called a hydatidiform mole. Only an overgrown placenta grows when you have this problem, and there is no fetus; so these cases always miscarry, but they are only seen in about 1 in 2,000 pregnancies. The diagnosis is easily made by a sonogram. For most women, the nausea and vomiting are over by the third or fourth month of pregnancy.

## Spitting

17. QUESTION: I keep spitting lots of saliva since I got pregnant. Does this mean an abnormal pregnancy and that miscarriage is likely?

ANSWER: Not at all. This condition is called hyperptyalism and usually means you have lots of normal hormones.

## Obesity

**18. QUESTION:** My doctor says I am obese. It took me a long time to get pregnant, and I am worried about miscarrying because of being obese.

**ANSWER:** Obese means that you are 30 percent or more above the average weight for your height. Obese women have a statistically greater chance of miscarrying, but so do very thin women. There are greater risks in pregnancy, as well, when you are obese. These include preterm births, gestational diabetes, hypertension, and Cesarean births. Despite these risks, pregnancy is not the right time to go on a weight-loss diet. If you can stay on a weight-control program during pregnancy, you will lose 25 to 30 pounds after giving birth. However, the best time to lose weight is before you become pregnant, and it will make it easier for you to conceive.

## LIFESTYLE QUESTIONS

### Raw Food

**19. QUESTION:** I like sushi. Can I eat it without worrying about miscarriage?

**ANSWER:** Uncooked food can make you sick but will not cause miscarriage if you are not ill to start with. Proper hydration and a call to your doctor for specific advice if you get food poisoning should prevent any serious consequences. Sushi without raw fish is safe. With raw fish you are at risk for food poisoning and tapeworm. However, a miscarriage is very unlikely unless there is a contaminant, such as listeria, a kind of bacteria known to be a cause of miscarriage.

### Weight Loss

**20. QUESTION:** My friend says that if I do not eat enough when I get pregnant and I lose weight instead of gaining, I could lose the baby.

**ANSWER:** Losing weight is common in the first two or three months because many women lose their appetite and do not eat much. The babies do just fine. Losing weight in pregnancy will normally result in a smaller than average baby, but not a miscarriage. A weight-loss program or a banding procedure for weight loss are best reserved for nonpregnant women, however.

## Medicines

21. QUESTION: I have been taking thyroid pills every day and now my home pregnancy test is positive. Should I stop them because I have been told that you should not take medicines when you are pregnant because it could cause a miscarriage or harm the baby?

ANSWER: You should call your doctor and ask about the medication that you are taking. In this case, stopping the medication would be more likely to cause harm than staying on it. Each medication is different for each person and should be discussed with your doctor before you get pregnant.

## Drugs

22. QUESTION: I smoked a couple of joints before I missed my period. Will that cause a miscarriage?

ANSWER: Using drugs in early pregnancy, once or twice, is unlikely to cause miscarriage. Continued use may damage your fetus, and certain drugs, like cocaine, can cause miscarriages even used only once and even later on in pregnancy.

## Alcohol

23. QUESTION: For the last few years I have one vodka martini before dinner to relax. My pregnancy test just came up positive, so do I have to stop?

ANSWER: Yes. In fact, the previous two weeks of alcohol probably have not increased your risk for miscarriage or an abnormal baby, but we do not know that for sure. The exact dose and timing of alcohol exposure that is harmful is not the same for everyone, but the damage is worse with more exposure. Do not drink if you plan pregnancy. An occasional sip of wine is not likely to cause a miscarriage, but the dose that may cause fetal damage, such as a learning disability, is not known.

## Folic Acid

24. QUESTION: Do I have to take folic acid pills in order to stay pregnant?

ANSWER: Folic acid is added to breads, cereals, and products like noodles and spaghetti by federal law in the United States. When you see the words "fortified" or "enriched," this means that folic acid has been added to the product. You do not need folic acid pills to avoid miscarriage, although there is some evidence that patients with a low level of folic acid have more pregnancy losses. Folic acid is most important in avoiding brain and spinal cord defects in the child. It should be taken before you get pregnant and through the first three months of pregnancy at least.

## Not Gaining Weight

25. QUESTION: My mother says that if I do not gain enough weight for the first three months of pregnancy, I could miscarry. Is that true?

ANSWER: Most women do not gain in the first month or two and will not miscarry. The amount of your weight gain is not related to miscarriage.

## Massage

26. QUESTION: Will having a massage make me miscarry?

ANSWER: There is no evidence that the usual massage techniques will cause miscarriage. However, I advise against vigorous massage of the abdomen based on studies of fetal injury in Pacific Islanders using birth massage techniques.

## Exercise

27. QUESTION: I work out with two hours of cardio and weights every day and I run three miles every other day. Will that cause a miscarriage?

ANSWER: Vigorous exercise has not been shown to cause a miscarriage. However, physical fitness is different from training to compete, and during a pregnancy your body will do 40 to 60 percent more work than in non-pregnancy given the same level of exercise. Ask your doctor or midwife about how much exercise is best for you.

## Tub Baths

28. QUESTION: Will taking a bath in a tub cause a miscarriage?
ANSWER: No. That is an old wives' tale.

## Hot Tubs, Whirlpools, and Jacuzzis

29. QUESTION: Will a whirlpool hot tub cause a miscarriage?
ANSWER: Hot tubs can raise your body temperature and will increase your pulse and the fetal heartbeat. The effects on the fetus are not known, but have not been associated with miscarriage. I advise against hot tubs because they may cause fainting in pregnant women.

## Saunas and Steam Baths

30. QUESTION: Can steam baths or saunas cause a miscarriage?
ANSWER: Like hot tubs, steam and sauna bathing raise your pulse, your core body temperature, and the fetal heart rate. I do not advise them in pregnancy, but they have not been associated with miscarriage.

## Sex in Pregnancy

31. QUESTION: My husband will not come near me because he thinks that sex will cause a miscarriage. Is he right?
ANSWER: He is wrong, but it is a common belief; however, there is no evidence that supports the idea. There are even some cultures that believe that sex is necessary to provide satisfactory nourishment for the fetus!

## Orgasm

32. QUESTION: My friend says that sex in pregnancy is okay, as long as the woman does not climax. Can climaxing cause a miscarriage?

ANSWER: The medical literature shows that there may be uterine contractions when a woman climaxes, but this does not lead to miscarriage. Multiple climaxes in a short time frame late in pregnancy might lead to preterm labor, but this has never been proven. There is insufficient published medical data on this subject. Nevertheless, many doctors advise against multiple partners and frequent intercourse in the last three months of pregnancy.

### Timing Pregnancy After Miscarriage

33. QUESTION: How long do I have to wait after miscarrying before I try again?

ANSWER: Many doctors disagree on when, but I tell my patients to wait for two or three cycles. I believe that this allows the lining of the uterus to grow back completely and the ovulation cycle to be restored to normal.

### Working

34. QUESTION: Will I have to quit my job as a waitress now that I am pregnant?

ANSWER: For most jobs, continued working in the absence of any symptoms of a threatened miscarriage is just fine. Pregnancy loss has been related to night work, and possibly to working more than eight hours a day seven days a week on your feet. Unless you own the restaurant or do frequent double shifts, most waitresses or other workers just do not work that hard. Check with your midwife or doctor about your work schedule when you are pregnant.

### Hair Dye

35. QUESTION: Will dyeing my hair cause a miscarriage or an abnormal baby?

ANSWER: There is insufficient medical evidence to support an increased miscarriage rate or fetal damage from dyeing your hair monthly during pregnancy. I advise my patients to go ahead and dye their hair. Even women who work dyeing other people's hair do not show a significant increased risk of miscarriage when all the other factors are considered.

## Nails
36. QUESTION: Will a manicure or pedicure increase my risk of miscarriage because of chemicals in the nail polish, nail polish remover, wraps, or glues?
ANSWER: No, you cannot absorb enough to do any harm.

## Coffee
37. QUESTION: Will drinking coffee cause a miscarriage?
ANSWER: There is minimal evidence showing a relationship between more than four cups a day and a higher frequency of miscarriage. I tell my patients that up to two cups is safe.

## Soda
38. QUESTION: Will drinking soda or diet soda make me lose my baby?
ANSWER: Neither has been shown to cause miscarriage. However, the diet additives NutraSweet, Splenda, and Sweet'N Low have not been fully studied in pregnancy.

## Sunscreen
39. QUESTION: Is it safe to use sunscreen lotion when you are pregnant?
ANSWER: There is no evidence that the usual suntan lotions can cause a miscarriage, but there are no adequate medical studies. Ask your doctor or midwife. My feeling is that not enough could be absorbed to have any meaningful effect.

## Mold
40. QUESTION: Mold was found in my house. Can it cause me to miscarry?

ANSWER: Exposure to mold can cause symptoms and, although rarely, even lung infections, but it has not been shown to increase the risk of miscarriage.

### Air Pollution

41. QUESTION: I live in a city with constant air pollution. Am I more likely to have a miscarriage?

ANSWER: Air pollution is a health hazard, but is not known to cause miscarriage.

### Allergy

42. QUESTION: I have lots of allergies. I worry that the medicine I take or an allergy attack could make me lose the baby.

ANSWER: Most allergies will not cause miscarriage. Severe asthma, or allergic shock (anaphylaxis in medical terms) might cause a pregnancy loss, but that is extremely rare. See your doctor before pregnancy to find out what to do about your allergies.

### Special Diets

43. QUESTION: I have celiac disease and have to be on a gluten-free diet. Does the lack of a normal diet increase my miscarriage risk?

ANSWER: Not at all. You should be on prenatal vitamins and take in enough calories, and that is perfectly fine.

### Travel

44. QUESTION: My mother says that traveling on a plane could cause a miscarriage. Is it okay?

ANSWER: There is no reason to think that air travel can cause miscarriages; however, the first three months of pregnancy is when most miscarriages occur. You would not want to have a problem on a plane, or be forced to have emergency treatment in an unknown place. That is why most doctors advise against travel by plane in the first trimester and in the last month or so of pregnancy. Even if you drive or take a train, you should get up and walk around every hour or two to improve blood circulation and prevent blood clot formation in your legs whenever you are pregnant and probably even if you are not pregnant.

## *Douching*

45. QUESTION: Will douching cause a miscarriage?

ANSWER: Most doctors advise against douching in pregnancy because of the remote possibility that the fluid could enter the uterus and cause infection or enough irritation to cause a miscarriage. There is not enough evidence to be sure, so it is best to avoid douching during pregnancy just to be on the safe side.

# MEDICAL INTERVENTION QUESTIONS

## *Amniocentesis*

46. QUESTION: My doctor says that I need an amniocentesis, but I am scared that I could lose the baby.

ANSWER: Amniocentesis done with ultrasound guidance has a miscarriage rate of one to three per thousand. The procedure is 99.9 percent accurate.

## *Chorionic Villus Sampling*

47. QUESTION: My doctor advised a CVS procedure because of my history of miscarriages. Will the procedure increase my risk for another miscarriage?

ANSWER: The CVS procedure carries a risk of 1 to 3 percent for miscarriage. This is minimally above the spontaneous miscarriage rate at the time that it is usually done, which is 10 to 13 weeks of pregnancy. You should discuss this with your doctor and follow what appears to you to be the best advice.

## Smoking

**48. QUESTION:** I smoke only two or three cigarettes a day. Do I have to stop?

**ANSWER:** It is not likely that it would cause a miscarriage, but it will decrease the weight of your baby. It would be best if you quit.

**49. QUESTION:** My husband smokes a lot. Could his smoking cause me to lose the baby?

**ANSWER:** There is insufficient information to answer but it seems very unlikely. Secondary smoke will increase your long-term health risks, but the effects on pregnancy are not known.

## Birth Control Pills

**50. QUESTION:** I stopped taking the birth control pill and got pregnant in that first cycle. Is that why I miscarried?

**ANSWER:** There are some data suggesting that the miscarriage rate is increased if pregnancy occurs immediately after stopping birth control pills. The presumption is that ovulation may not be synchronized with proper development of the lining of the uterus. That may interfere with the normal process of implantation and lead to pregnancy loss. The medical evidence for this is sparse, but I ask my patients to wait for two menstrual cycles before trying for this reason.

## Non-hormonal Contraceptives

**51. QUESTION:** How long do I wait after I discontinue using condoms? How long after the diaphragm? How long after using a spermicide by itself or with these?

**ANSWER:** You need not wait at all. The next cycle would be fine.

## Intrauterine Device

**52. QUESTION:** How long should I wait after taking out an intrauterine device in order to avoid miscarrying?

**ANSWER:** The medical evidence is limited, so I generally advise two menstrual cycles to enable the inflammation in the uterus, due to the IUD, to clear up.

## IUD in Place

**53. QUESTION:** I just found out that I am pregnant, and I still have my IUD. What do I do now, because I am worried that I will miscarry?

**ANSWER:** First you need an exam and a sonogram to see if the IUD is indeed still there, and secondly to exclude an ectopic pregnancy. (See Chapter 11.) Next, if it is still there, at that visit the IUD should be removed if the string is accessible. The risk of miscarriage is not as bad if the IUD is removed, but it is still somewhat increased. If it cannot be removed, the risks of miscarriage and infection are also increased, but a normal-term birth is still possible. You need to have a full discussion with your doctor and come to a decision about that.

## Dental Work

**54. QUESTION:** I want to get my dental work done, but I am afraid that it could cause a miscarriage. Do I have to suffer with the pain for the whole pregnancy?

**ANSWER:** Dental work, both emergency and maintenance, does not cause miscarriage. Pregnancy tends to cause gum bleeding, and proper dental care may even help to avoid preterm labor. You may see your dentist and get appropriate treatment.

## X-Rays

**55. QUESTION:** My dentist wants me to take X-rays, but I am worried that it could cause harm to the baby or even a miscarriage.

**ANSWER:** Dental X-rays or even chest X-rays or CT scans will not cause miscarriage, and the dose is too low to harm the baby. However, X-rays are cumulative in that their effects keep on adding up throughout your life. Avoiding them, if possible, is sensible, and exposing your fetus starts your child off with its first dose. Fortunately, lead aprons will shield the fetus when a dental or chest X-ray is necessary. Consult with your doctor when being advised to have an X-ray.

## Assisted Reproductive Technologies

56. QUESTION: When I became pregnant by in vitro fertilization, I was started on progesterone injections because they said that I had a higher risk of miscarriage. Is that true?

ANSWER: Early pregnancy loss in the first trimester, including ectopic pregnancy, is more frequent than in spontaneous pregnancy; however, it still adds up to only about one-third of the embryo transfers on the average, more in older women.

## Progesterone

57. QUESTION: Does progesterone treatment prevent miscarriage?

ANSWER: Progesterone can prevent miscarriage due to an inadequate corpus luteum. (See Chapter 17.) The corpus luteum is usually the main source of progesterone in early pregnancy up until the tenth week. When it is not functioning well, the progesterone level is too low, and giving progesterone may salvage a pregnancy that is otherwise normal, but would be lost. A defective embryo will not be saved and miscarriage will follow, so an abnormal fetus cannot be preserved by progesterone therapy.

## Sonograms

58. QUESTION: Can a sonogram cause a miscarriage?

ANSWER: Sonograms of various kinds have been done on millions of women over the last 35 years with no credible evidence for increased risk of miscarriage.

## Internal Examination

59. QUESTION: Can an internal pelvic examination cause a miscarriage?

ANSWER: There is no evidence to suggest that a pelvic examination can cause a miscarriage. Sometimes, a pelvic examination, or a Pap test, can cause bleeding from the very soft tissues of the cervix in pregnancy, which can bleed much more easily than when not pregnant. That bleeding is just from the mouth of the womb, and not from the pregnancy. It usually is not heavy, stops in three days or so, and does not involve any increased risk of pregnancy loss. Only when the placenta is lying over the cervix (placenta previa) can a pelvic exam cause heavy bleeding. Even then, pregnancy loss is uncommon.

## Breast Fullness

60. QUESTION: My breasts felt full and sensitive, and now I do not feel that they are like that anymore. Is that a sign that the pregnancy is failing?

ANSWER: Usually, that is a normal variation and does not mean that anything bad is happening. Sometimes, it does occur along with increasing cramps and bleeding, and that can mean a threatened miscarriage. See your doctor or midwife if you are having all of these symptoms. It is possible to offer treatment for certain kinds of threatened miscarriage, or you may find out that the symptoms are not causing a miscarriage.

## Vaginal Creams

61. QUESTION: Can I use a vaginal cream without causing a miscarriage?

ANSWER: Most vaginal creams and lubricants can be used in pregnancy without causing miscarriage. Check with your doctor or midwife before using one to be sure about any possible other effects.

# GLOSSARY

ABC ⁓ An easy mnemonic device to remember the main symptoms of a threatened miscarriage: A for abdominal pain, B for bleeding, and C for cramps.

ADHESIONS ⁓ Attachment of tissues and adjacent structures to each other by scars.

AMNIOCENTESIS ⁓ A procedure through which a long needle is passed into the pregnant uterus through the mother's abdomen and a sample of the fluid around the baby is drawn off to be tested. Chromosomes and many illnesses can be looked for as well as fetal lung maturity.

ANTICARDIOLIPIN ANTIBODIES ⁓ A form of phospholipid antibody that resembles a component used in a standard blood test for syphilis.

ANTINUCLEAR ANTIBODY (ANA) ⁓ The ANA is a blood test that is often positive in patients with auto-immune diseases; the level rises as the disease gets worse.

ANTIPHOSPHOLIPID SYNDROME ⁓ An auto-immune condition in which antiphospholipid antibodies are markers of disease in which a patient's immune system attacks her own cells and will attack cells in her placenta and fetus.

ASHERMAN SYNDROME ⁓ The problem of scar tissue (intrauterine adhesions) inside the uterus as a cause of repeated miscarriages.

ASYMMETRICAL UTERINE SEPTUM ⁓ When the uterus is divided into two unequal parts with a small channel between them.

AUTO-IMMUNE DISEASE ⁓ The body's immune system is hardwired to create antibodies to fight off foreign invaders that enter the body and threaten to upset the status quo. Normally, this is a good thing—your own personal army defending you against attackers. Sometimes, however, the immune system misinterprets good cells as foreign entities, attacking them and causing ailments resulting from that fight. In the case of auto-immune disease and pregnancy, the mother's and the fetus's immune systems are communicating with each other and the mother creates anti-bodies against her own cells. These antibodies get into the placenta (after-birth), which is the organ that supports and protects the growing fetus, and can affect the placenta and the fetus to cause damage and miscarriage. The placenta and fetus share certain cell markers (antigens) with the mother and these are attacked by maternal auto-antibodies. The disease that makes your own body attack itself makes a pregnant woman's im-mune system attack the similar markers on the placenta and fetus, half of which come from the mother and half from the father.

BALANCED CHROMOSOME DEFECT — An abnormal arrangement of chromosomes in which a missing piece of one is attached to another so that the total material is normal. This is referred to as a process of translocation, because the DNA-carrying segment is now in the wrong place. The person is normal, but the sperm or egg may carry too much or too little genetic material, because a sperm or an egg carries only half the chromosomes. If the half has the extra piece, there is too much; if it car-ries the chromosome with the missing piece, it is too little.

BICORNUATE UTERUS — Two separated bodies of the uterus, each one-half of a uterus with one tube and one ovary attached to each half.

BIOPHYSICAL PROFILE — A combination of ultrasound and fetal heart rate monitoring to evaluate the fetal heartbeat, breathing, and body movements, as well as the amount of amniotic fluid present. If there is too little amniotic fluid, the risk of losing the baby is greater.

BLIGHTED OVUM — An outdated and often inaccurate term used to describe an abnormal ovum, or egg, as cause for an unhealthy pregnancy instead of an abnormal embryo as cause for miscarriage.

BLOOD HORMONE LEVELS — Measurements of the concentration of hormones in a blood sample. For example, your pregnancy blood hor-mones are: chorionic gonadotropin, progesterone, and estradiol. These pregnancy hormones usually rise throughout the first three months of pregnancy. When that is not happening, miscarriage is more likely to occur.

BREECH ⁓ When the baby is positioned in the mother's womb with the bottom facing toward the vagina, so that it will come out of the mother feet- or behind first.

BREECH EXTRACTION ⁓ A breech baby is delivered feetfirst by a series of obstetrical maneuvers very different from the way a normal head-first delivery is done.

BRUCELLOSIS ⁓ A bacterial infection with the *Brucella* bacteria, which can cause miscarriage.

CERCLAGE OPERATION ⁓ The two basic cerclage operations are the MacDonald and the Shirodkar, named after the physicians who first described them. During a MacDonald cerclage procedure, a band of strong thread is stitched through the weakened cervix and tightened until the cervix is firmly shut, like a purse string. The thread is generally removed around 37 weeks of pregnancy. The Shirodkar operation uses a wide band under the skin of the cervix to lengthen and narrow the opening. The doctor can remove the band in labor or at about 37 weeks, as well.

CERVICAL CONIZATION ⁓ Also referred to as a cone biopsy or cold knife cone biopsy, cervical conization is used for diagnosis and/or treatment of pre-cancerous cervical conditions. A cone-shaped piece of the cervix is removed, usually accompanied by a D&C. This can be accomplished by using a scalpel (cold knife), a laser, or a cautery electrode (a LEEP, pronounces like "leap," or LLETZ, pronounces like "let's").

CERVIX ⁓ The part of the uterus (womb) that protrudes into the top of the vagina and has an opening into the uterus. It is often referred to as the mouth of the womb.

CHORIONIC VILLUS SAMPLING (CVS) ⁓ A genetic test performed at 10 to 12 weeks of pregnancy where a minuscule piece of the placenta is biopsied in order to detect abnormalities with a fetus early on.

CLOMIPHENE ⁓ A drug to induce the pituitary gland to release follicle-stimulating hormone (FSH), a hormone secreted by the pituitary gland that causes the ovary to ripen eggs to be ovulated.

**COMPLEMENT** — Part of the immune system, which is often abnormal in the blood of patients with auto-immune disease, especially with systemic lupus.

**CORPUS LUTEUM** — The corpus luteum is the part of the ovary that secretes the hormones that support early pregnancy after ovulation. When pregnancy does not occur and the hormone levels from the corpus luteum begin to fade, menstruation follows.

**CORTISOL** — A hormone released by the adrenal glands, which is a key hormone for helping your body react to and handle stress and which aids in the breakdown of food for energy. It is released from the glands into the blood and excreted in urine.

**CYTOMEGALOVIRUS (CMV)** — Causes a mild respiratory illness in most patients and is barely noticed, but may infect a fetus when it is the mom's first encounter with the virus and cause miscarriage.

**DEHYDROEPIANDROSTERONE (DHEA)** — A male hormone produced by the adrenal glands in men and women. It is usually present in small amounts in women.

**DIABETES** — A disease that affects the way the body uses food. It is caused by a lack of insulin, a hormone made in the pancreas that is essential for converting energy from food. Insulin is necessary for the body to process nutrients (carbohydrates, fats, and proteins), and its absence causes high sugar (glucose) levels in the blood.

**DIETHYLSTILBESTROL (DES)** — Diethylstilbestrol is a synthetic form of estrogen that was used to prevent miscarriage and treat diabetes in the U.S. between 1938 and 1971. Medical follow-up by Dr. Arthur Herbst of children exposed in the womb found that it sometimes caused vaginal cancer, and often caused abnormalities of the reproductive system and incompetent cervix in female children exposed to it. Exposed boys may also suffer damage to their reproductive system.

**DILATION AND CURETTAGE (D&C)** — A D&C is a procedure in which the cervical passageway is opened (dilation) and the uterine lining is scraped (curettage).

DISCORDANT TWINS — Twins that differ from each other by at least 20 percent in weight. This can be accompanied by differences in gender, abnormalities, or placentas.

DOPPLER STUDY — An ultrasound technique to measure blood flow used for the umbilical artery or the middle cerebral artery to determine the blood flow between the fetus and placenta or the blood flow in the baby's brain.

ECTOPIC PREGNANCY — When a fertilized egg implants itself outside of the uterine walls, and settles in the fallopian tube (tubal pregnancy, the most common form of ectopic pregnancy), ovary, abdomen, or cervix, the pregnancy is considered ectopic. The organ where the fetus has implanted itself eventually bursts as the fetus grows, causing severe bleeding, which is potentially life threatening.

ENDOMETRIOSIS — The lining of the womb is growing outside the womb, often on the ovaries, oviducts, and in the spaces between them, the back of the womb, and the intestines. This can interfere with the function of the fallopian tubes and prevent fertilization, leading to infertility.

ENDOMETRIUM — The tissue lining the uterus.

ENDOSCOPY — Using a telescopic instrument to visualize structures within the body.

ENZYME — A protein that acts to cause a chemical reaction to go forward quickly.

EPIDURAL ANESTHESIA — A method of numbing the pelvic nerves by inserting a catheter via a needle in the space between the vertebrae and spinal cord (called the epidural space). Injection of the anesthetic drug through the catheter permits continuous release of anesthesia.

ESTRADIOL — The major female hormone, an essential component of female physiology.

FACTOR V LEIDEN — This mutation is a genetic condition that predisposes a mother to abnormal clot formation in the blood vessels. When it affects the placenta, it leads to pregnancy loss in some cases.

FALLOPIAN TUBES — Also called oviducts, these are the flexible, moving structures that carry the released eggs, or ova, from the ovaries to the uterus.

**FETAL ALCOHOL SYNDROME** — The resulting birth defects caused by severe alcohol abuse by a pregnant mother, which include neurological abnormalities, growth retardation, developmental disabilities, and physical abnormalities.

**FETOSCOPIC LASER SURGERY** — Using a tiny endoscope to operate inside a pregnant uterus with lasers. This coagulates the communicating blood vessels connecting the twins' blood flow in the placenta that is shared by the two fetuses. This separates their blood circulations from each other in an attempt to save both twins.

**FIBROIDS** — A benign tumor of the uterus, which arises from muscle cells but looks fibrous when cut open.

**FORTIFIED** — The addition of essential nutrients to a food, regardless of whether that nutrient is normally contained in the food, for the purpose of improving the diet.

**FSH** — Follicle-stimulating hormone (FSH) is secreted by the pituitary gland and causes the ovary to ripen eggs to be ovulated.

**GENE** — The specific package of DNA on a chromosome that directs a cell to make a specific protein.

**GONADOTROPIN THERAPY** — Injections of a hormone or combination of hormones to stimulate the ovaries to make eggs.

**HCG** — Human chorionic gonadotropin (HCG) is a hormone produced by the growing placenta.

**HORMONES** — Chemical messengers produced by special cells in your body's organs. These organs are called glands. The hormones are released into your blood and regulate specific targets like your ovaries, blood vessels, kidneys, and other structures throughout the body.

**HYDATIDIFORM MOLE** — A precancerous condition of the placenta, which will require a dilation and curettage (D&C) and sometimes a course of chemotherapy. This disease can be diagnosed by the sonogram and is usually detectable by the end of the first trimester at the latest. Sometimes it can be missed until the tissue is examined under the microscope. The hydatidiform mole can be cured almost 100 percent of the time by appropriate treatment if diagnosed early.

HYPERTHYROIDISM — The medical term for an overactive thyroid.

HYSTEROGRAM — A picture of the uterus usually made by X-ray or fluoroscopic imaging of the uterus after dye has been injected into it through the cervix. When it includes the oviducts it is called a hystero-salpingogram.

HYSTEROSALPINGOGRAM — A radiopaque dye solution is slowly injected into the uterus through a tube placed in the cervix vaginally. X-rays are taken, producing pictures that will outline the inside of the cervix, uterus, and fallopian tubes. They demonstrate that the tubes are not closed off to the uterus or the ovaries and show what the inside of the uterus looks like.

HYSTEROSCOPY — After opening the cervix as is normally done in a D&C, a fiber-optic telescope with channels for inserting tiny instruments is attached to a small TV camera and inserted into the uterus to view the cavity and perform surgery as necessary.

IMPLANTATION — A process by which the embryo buries itself in the lining of the uterus.

INCOMPETENT CERVIX — In pregnancy, the cervix, which is made up mostly of fibrous tissue, does not open until labor begins and the baby is ready to be born. However, sometimes a cervix may have been weak-ened due to congenital or other factors, such as tearing in childbirth or trauma from an abortion, causing it to open long before a fetus is ready to be born and often resulting in miscarriage during the second trimester.

INTERSTITIAL PREGNANCY — An ectopic pregnancy that develops in the uterine, or interstitial, section of the fallopian tube.

IN VITRO FERTILIZATION (IVF) — In vitro means "glass" in Latin, so, literally, the procedure means "by fertilization in glass." After using injec-tions to stimulate the ovaries and make many eggs, the eggs are removed from the ovaries and fertilized with the man's sperm outside the body in a glass container. The fertilized eggs are examined under a microscope, and the healthiest looking of these embryos are then introduced into the woman's uterus through a fine tube placed into her cervix vaginally.

LAPAROSCOPIC SURGERY — Considered a minimally invasive pro-cedure, laparoscopic surgery is performed by making several small incisions in the abdomen, usually one-half to one centimeter in length. An incision is made through the navel (although the incision may also be made just below the navel, I like to make it through the navel so the scar can't be seen). A thin, long tube called a laparoscope is inserted through the incision into the patient. A camera is attached to the outside of the laparoscope, enabling the surgeon to see inside the patient by viewing an image on a TV screen transmitted by the camera. Tiny instruments are then inserted through secondary incisions to perform the surgery.

L/S RATIO — A test done on amniotic fluid in which the chemicals lecithin and sphingomyelin are measured, and the ratio of the lecithin (L) to the sphingomyelin (S) is calculated. When the fetal lungs are producing enough surfactant, a chemical that keeps them open, the lungs are believed to be mature. The L/S ratio is an indicator of how much surfactant is present in the fetus, since lecithin is a component of surfactant and sphingomyelin is usually present in a steady amount throughout pregnancy.

LUTEAL PHASE — The luteal phase is the 14 days from the time of ovulation to the beginning of menstruation.

LUTEAL PHASE DEFICIENCY — The luteal phase is the 14 days from the time of ovulation to the beginning of menstruation. A lack of sufficient hormones to support an early pregnancy is a luteal phase deficiency. This happens when there is an inadequate corpus luteum producing an inadequate amount of progesterone.

LYMPHEDEMA — The lymph system is in part responsible for "filtering" the fluid that surrounds your cells. With lymphedema a buildup of fluid occurs in the lymphatic system, which causes swelling and discomfort and, at worst, greater susceptibility to infection. While there can be other causes of lymphedema, it is not uncommon in breast cancer patients who have had lymph nodes removed with the cancer as part of their treatment.

METABOLISM — The chemical processes by which your body uses the food you eat as fuel to drive all of the body's functions.

MOLAR PREGNANCY — The placenta is abnormal with excessive growth leading to hydatidiform mole. There is no fetus or rarely there is a fetus present, but molar pregnancy always results in a miscarriage. Hydatidiform mole occurs about 1 in 2,000 pregnancies and can go on to choriocarcinoma, a type of cancer, in about 1 percent of molar pregnancies.

MONOZYGOTIC (IDENTICAL) TWINS — Twins that come from a single fertilized egg and are almost always mirror images of each other. Their placentas are fused, but they can vary in the amount of blood supply per twin, as well as weight or abnormalities.

MULTIFETAL PREGNANCY REDUCTION — Partial abortion of one or more fetuses, preserving the rest in order to continue the pregnancy and decrease the risk of preterm births.

MYCOPLASMAS — A rare type of infecting bacteria-like organism that can cause miscarriage.

MYOMECTOMY — An operation to remove a fibroid or fibroids.

NONSTRESS TEST — A fetal heart rate test to evaluate fetal well-being by observing increases in the fetal heart rate associated with fetal movements.

NUTRACEUTICAL — A food or part of a food or food supplement that may provide medical or general health benefits. It is often a natural product, such as garlic, or it may be a specific component of a food, such as the omega-3s in fish oil, or it may be a natural product with no specific basis for activity as a food supplement.

OVARIAN FOLLICLE — A roundish cavity that contains fluid and a maturing egg, or ovum, and is surrounded by a layer of cells.

OVARIAN HYPERSTIMULATION SYNDROME (OHSS) — OHSS occurs when drugs used to induce ovulation cause rapid enlargement of the ovarian cysts and fluid accumulates in them, as well as inside the abdominal cavity. This causes a drop in the patient's circulating blood volume and may lead to low blood pressure and shock.

OVARIAN TORSION — The ovary and usually the oviduct twist, and their blood supply gets blocked, often causing severe abdominal pain and death of the ovary and oviduct.

OVULATION — The midway point during the menstrual cycle when a mature egg, or ovum, is released from an ovary and sent down the fallopian tube (oviduct) into the uterus. If fertilization does not occur, the egg will be absorbed. Although most menstrual cycles are based on a 28-day calendar, many women have shorter or longer cycles, and thus ovulation can occur earlier or later than the standard midpoint of day 14 to 16. Every month the cycle is started by hormones that stimulate about 20 of the 300,000 or so eggs stored in your ovaries. Usually, only one egg develops enough to respond to the hormonal trigger to ovulate, while the other 19 break down and get absorbed. Once the egg and sperm meet in the oviduct and unite in fertilization, the embryo begins to form as it journeys to the uterus. That trip takes about three days and then the embryo attaches itself to the wall of the uterus. This is implantation, as the embryo buries itself in the lining tissues of the uterus and is nourished there.

PCBS — Polychlorinated biphenyls (PCBs) are synthetic compounds that are the poisonous leftovers from toxic industrial chemicals, which were banned in the United States in 1977. However, PCBs still exist in many areas of the environment, and are commonly found in the bottom of rivers and lakes. They build up in the fatty tissue of certain fish and, although are not known to be generally harmful in small doses to the average person, they can cause birth defects and possibly miscarriage if consumed in large quantities.

PELVIC INFLAMMATORY DISEASE (PID) — PID is an infection often caused by sexually transmitted organisms (most often chlamydia or gonorrhea), affecting a woman's reproductive organs. Symptoms of PID include fever, painful urination, painful intercourse, irregular menstrual bleeding, and an odorous vaginal discharge. Sometimes symptoms are mild and may go away quickly, but the damage to the tubes may still occur. Rarely, a sore throat or respiratory infection may enter the bloodstream and land in the tubes, causing PID from a non–sexually transmitted source.

PLACENTA — The afterbirth, which is an organ of fetal origin that grows into the mother's uterine wall for its blood supply and provides oxygen and nutrition to the fetus while removing fetal carbon dioxide and products of fetal metabolism.

PLACENTA ACCRETA — The placenta is attached so deeply in the wall of the uterus that it cannot separate normally and when the pregnancy is over, attempts to separate the placenta will result in severe hemorrhage, usually requiring hysterectomy to save the life of the woman.

PLACENTA PREVIA — The placenta, or afterbirth, is coming first, ahead of the baby and lying over the mouth of the womb. When there are uterine contractions this location of the placenta provides for very poor attachment to the wall of the uterus and the result is bleeding, which is sometimes very heavy.

PLATELET ANTIBODIES — The pregnant woman makes antibodies against the blood platelets. This occurs when the platelets contain a factor contributed by the father that is absent in the mother's blood. The result is destruction of the fetal blood platelets, which causes fetal bleeding and death of the fetus in the uterus or in labor.

POLYCYSTIC OVARY SYNDROME (PCO) — A condition in which the ovaries are enlarged and filled with fluid cysts and do not ovulate. There is a high degree of male hormone present and the patient is often overweight and infertile.

PREIMPLANTATION GENETIC DIAGNOSIS (PGD) — A program of in vitro fertilization is begun, and multiple eggs are fertilized in the laboratory. Then, several embryos, at three days past fertilization, when they consist of only six to eight cells, are selected. One cell, of the six or eight, is removed from the embryo, and the chromosomes are checked. The embryo does not even notice the missing cell, so if it has normal chromosomes, the embryo is transferred to the prepared uterus and a normal baby is likely if all other things remain normal.

PRETERM RUPTURE OF THE MEMBRANES (PROM) — The membranes, the sac filled with amniotic fluid in which the fetus floats, burst before labor begins. This occurs at times in patients where bacteria can ascend into the cervix and reach the membrane around the baby. If the bacteria create a serious infection, the mom may develop a fever and go into premature labor.

PROGESTERONE SUPPOSITORIES — A suppository that is inserted vaginally. Once inside the vagina, it softens and releases progesterone into a mother's body. This is used when it is necessary to augment inadequate progesterone production, a hormone that must be present at certain levels during the first ten weeks in order to ensure the continuation of a pregnancy. Not all pharmacies have the capability to make them, so if they are prescribed for you, be sure to check with your regular pharmacy first. Otherwise, ask your doctor if she has a list of pharmacies that provide them.

RECOMMENDED DIETARY ALLOWANCE (RDA) — The average daily intake that is sufficient to meet the nutritional requirements of nearly all healthy persons in each age and gender group, as well as in pregnancy.

RECURRENT ABORTION — The medical term for three miscarriages in a row, the point at which the statistical probability of another miscarriage increases from 25 to 28 percent. Some studies suggest a risk of up to 40 percent, but most of the medical information indicates about 28 percent is correct.

RECURRENT MISCARRIAGE — Having three or more instances of known pregnancy loss in a row.

RESECTOSCOPE — An instrument that can be passed through a hysteroscope and has an electrical loop, which allows for removal of tissue and coagulation to prevent bleeding at the same time.

RETROVERTED UTERUS — A condition in which a woman's uterus is tipped back toward the spine instead of forward toward the bladder.

RH FACTOR — Everyone has a blood type—A, B, AB, or O—which can be positive or negative. Your Rh factor is a marker (antigen) on your red blood cells that is either positive or negative. While most people (85 percent) are Rh positive, a small percentage are Rh negative.

SELECTIVE TERMINATION — Selective termination is a form of multifetal pregnancy reduction when there is one abnormal fetus, which can be aborted leaving the normal fetus to continue the pregnancy.

SEMINAL FLUID — The ejaculatory fluid that a man expels during sexual intercourse, which contains sperm.

SERIAL AMNIOCENTESIS — This procedure repeatedly removes excessive amniotic fluid (polyhydramnios) from the amniotic sac.

SHIRODKAR OPERATION — A procedure that corrects a weakened cervix by placing a woven band under the skin of a woman's cervix in order to support and reinforce the cervix. It is usually done no earlier than 12 weeks to make sure that there are no other causes of miscarriage in that pregnancy.

SONOGRAM — A picture made by computer analysis of sound waves reflected off an object, e.g., a baby inside its mother's womb. The process of getting the picture is called sonography, or ultrasonography.

SONOHYSTEROGRAM — A sterile solution is instilled vaginally through the cervix into the uterus and ultrasound pictures are taken to outline the uterus and the inside cavity of the uterus.

SUBCUTANEOUS INJECTION — An injection that is shot into the body just below the dermal and epidermal layers of skin into the subcutis layer.

SUPPLEMENT — An additional nutrient that may be added to your usual diet.

SYSTEMIC LUPUS ERYTHEMATOSUS — A generalized auto-immune disease that damages joints, skin, lungs, kidneys, and other organs.

THROMBOPHILIA — A blood-clotting disorder in which there is a tendency to excessive blood clotting under certain circumstances.

TOLERABLE UPPER INTAKE LEVEL (UL) — The maximum amount of a nutrient that can be taken on a daily basis, which poses no risk of an adverse effect on the health of the mother or baby.

UMBILICAL ARTERY DOPPLER BLOOD FLOW — A test using an ultrasound machine to evaluate the blood flow in the fetal umbilical artery in order to determine if it is getting enough blood flow through the placenta.

UMBILICAL CORD COAGULATION — If an abnormality is present in one twin, or that twin is already dying and cannot be saved, coagulating, or stopping the blood flow, in the umbilical cord of the abnormal twin will stop the transfusion process and prevent blood loss into a dead fetus from the healthy one, and thus save the life of the latter.

UNICORNUATE UTERUS — A condition when only one-half of the uterus is present.

UNPASTEURIZED — Pasteurization is the process, discovered by the French scientist Louis Pasteur, in which bacteria lurking in milk, other liquids, or cheese (prior to becoming a solid) are killed by heating the liquid to boiling temperature for at least 20 minutes. Foods not treated by this process are unpasteurized.

UTERINE SEPTUM — A growth of tissue down the center of the inside of the uterus that divides it into two separate halves.

UTERUS — The female reproductive organ to which the fallopian tubes and cervix are attached. Also called the womb, it carries the pregnancy.

VANISHING TWIN SYNDROME — The spontaneous loss of one embryo in a multiple pregnancy in the first three months. It usually disappears completely and is absorbed.

WOMB — The uterus; the female organ in which a baby grows.

# INDEX

*Page numbers of illustrations appear in italics.*

fetal monitoring (*cont.*)
 echocardiogram, 267, 271
 fetal kick counts, 267, 271
 heart rate (nonstress test), 166,
  203, 204, 271
 lung maturity, 167
 sonogram, 28, 38–39, 46, 122, 166,
  203, 222–23, 235, 266, 267, 271,
  272
 umbilical artery Doppler blood
  flow studies, 146, 147, 166, 183,
  184, 272
 well-being studies, 267
fetoscopic laser surgery, 151
fever, 87, 94, 123, 232, 233, 235, 238,
 246, 253, 289
fibroids, 57, 60, 116, 131–40
 birth control pills and, 131–32
 diagnosing, 137
 estrogen and progesterone
  receptors and, 134, 137
 as miscarriage risk factor, 113, 117,
  131–40
 pain and, 137
 preterm labor and, 137
 symptoms, 136
 treatment, 69, 133–36, 137–39
 vaginal vs. Cesarean birth
  following removal, 139–40
 what they are, 136–37
fine needle cautery, 128
first trimester of pregnancy
 abnormal fetus, as primary cause
  for miscarriage during, 53, 205
 antiphospholipid antibodies and
  miscarriage, 214
 blood-clotting disorders and
  miscarriage, 51, 57
 eating properly, 22
 lack of progesterone and
  miscarriage, xvi (*see also* luteal
  phase deficiency)
 miscarriages during, 27–28, 29, 42,
  53, 56, 104, 113, 117, 170, 197, 198,
  209, 233, 243
 nausea and loss of appetite, 22
folic acid
 anemia and, 18
 food sources, 12, 18–19, 22
 excess, and B$_{12}$ function, 12
 pre-conceptual supplements, 12
 prenatal supplements, 18–19

 reducing risk of fetal abnormalities
  and, 18, 293
food. *See* diet
food poisoning, 246, 251–53, 254,
 291
 when to call your doctor, 254
fright, 87
FSH (follicle stimulating hormone),
 45, 69, 244, 245
 testing, 49, 58, 64

**G**

genes, 205–6
genetic disorders/abnormality,
 197–208. *See also* abnormal
 embryo; empty sac (blighted
 ovum)
 chorionic villus sampling (CVS),
  154
 miscarriage and, 32
 Monosomy 21, xvi
 percentage of miscarriages from, 9
 testing for, 9–10
genetic screening, 4, 9–10
German measles. *See* rubella (German
 measles)
GIFT (gamete intrafallopian
 transfer), 69
gonadotropin therapy, 65, 69–70, 143,
 144
 multiple pregnancies and, 143–44
 risks of, 143
gonorrhea, 10
grieving, 277–80

**H**

hair dye/hair treatments, 82, 251, 254,
 295–96
heartburn, 22
hemolytic anemia, 51
hemophilia, 224
heparin, 51, 212, 215, 218, 222, 223,
 226
hepatitis
 A, 238
 B, 238
 testing for (hepatitis B surface
  antigen test), 10
herbal remedies and therapies, 249,
 253
Herbst, Arthur, 96, 124
herpes, 236, 238

# ABOUT THE AUTHORS

**Dr. Bruce Young** is internationally known as a leader and innovator in obstetrics and gynecology. He introduced many diagnostic and therapeutic modalities, which became standards of care in today's obstetrics and gynecology, and he was among the first to help women with serious medical conditions to have children. Most recently, he performed the first endoscopic fetal surgery in New York State and gained worldwide recognition for successful repair of preterm ruptured membranes to prevent pregnancy loss.

He founded the first maternal-fetal medicine program in the city of New York, the Division of Maternal-Fetal Medicine at NYU Medical Center. He has lectured worldwide and has earned numerous awards, including the March of Dimes Award for Distinguished Voluntary Service in Prevention of Birth Defects, the Distinguished Alumnus Award from the Department of Obstetrics and Gynecology at the NYU School of Medicine, the American College of Obstetricians and Gynecologists Award for Outstanding Achievement, and the Berson Award of the NYU School of Medicine for Achievement in Clinical Science. He has published over 100 research articles, more than a dozen scientific book chapters, and two perinatal medicine books. He is currently the Silverman Professor of Obstetrics and Gynecology at the New York University Medical Center. The NYU Department of Obstetrics and Gynecology Annual Research Day is named after him, and he is listed in *America's Top Doctors* and *New York Magazine*'s "Best Doctors" issue every year since their inception.

A graduate of New York University School of Journalism, **Amy Zavatto** is a freelance writer who lives in New York City. Her work appears in Planned Parenthood's Teenwire Web site, as well as *New York Magazine, Plenty, Gotham Magazine, Imbibe, Food & Wine,* and many others. Her fiction has appeared in *Jane* and she is the co-author of *The Renaissance Guide to Wine & Food Pairing.*